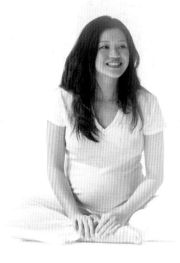

Dr. Jane MacDougall

PREGNANCY
WEEK BY WEEK

hamlyn

First published in Great Britain in 2011 by Caroll & Brown

This edition published in 2016 by Hamlyn,
a division of Octopus Publishing Group Ltd
Carmelite House
50 Victoria Embankment
London EC4Y 0DZ
www.octopusbooks.co.uk

A Hachette UK Company
www.hachette.co.uk

Distributed in the US by Hachette Book Group
1290 Avenue of the Americas, 4th and 5th Floors
New York, NY 10020

Distributed in Canada by Canadian Manda Group
664 Annette St., Toronto, Ontario, Canada M6S 2C8

ISBN 978 060063 221 4

Printed and bound in China

3 5 7 9 10 8 6 4 2

Illustrations
Amanda Williams

Suppliers
Thanks to Mothercare, for equipment shown p38, p54 (blankets),
and p56.

Photolibrary.com
Jacket, p6, p14, p20, p22, p42 bottom left, p62, p74, p76, p82, p87,
and p88.

Science Photo Library
P8 Prof. P. Motta/Dept. of Anatomy/University "La Sapienza,"
Rome/Science Photo Library and p22 Ian Hooton/Science
Photo Library.

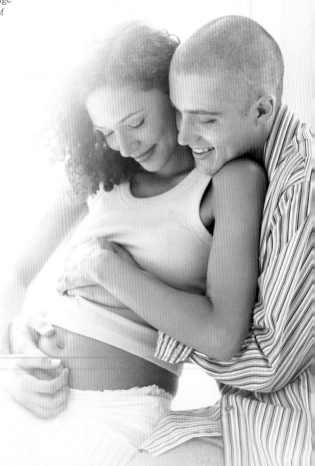

CONTENTS

FOREWORD

Pregnancy Week by Week is the best companion any expectant mother can have. Although every pregnancy is unique, the book covers the experiences most women are likely to have over these nine vital months, as well as showing how an unborn baby develops in the uterus from week to week. There is also a "dates for your diary" planner at the bottom of every week page on which to jot down your prenatal appointments, test dates and results, and to record any important tasks and events. This can help ensure both you and your baby's good health and help you prepare for your baby's arrival.

The book's convenient size means you can carry it around with you to your appointments—or when you are going out for any reason. Its spiral binding enables you to prop the book up on your dresser or desk, so that you can see at a glance the changes to your baby taking place each week, as well as your appointments diary, if you need to.

Inside you will find accurate and accessible information, reflecting current medical opinion on a variety of subjects ranging from preconception care, how to cope with common symptoms of pregnancy, nutritional and exercise advice, the latest medical and diagnostic tests, information on where and how to have your baby, what to pack for the hospital, and how to decorate your baby's nursery.

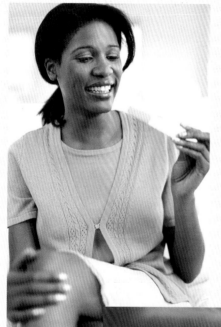

The text contains many headings and information boxes, which make it easy for you to dip in to find the subject you require, without needing to read the whole book cover to cover. Your baby's weekly progress is imagined in specially commissioned illustrations augmented by information on his probable size.

Pregnancy Week by Week is the ideal book to buy for yourself or for anyone else planning a family, and a great gift for those already expecting, as well as for prospective grandparents. It aims to provide concise, reassuring advice leading to a healthy and happy pregnancy and a healthy newborn—with the added satisfaction of being able to view the new baby's development.

USEFUL CONTACT DETAILS

As a quick and easy reference, fill in the following information and try to keep it as up to date as possible.

This book belongs to
Name

Address

Telephone number

Blood group

Allergies

Medications

Birth partner
Name

Telephone number

Hospital
Name

Address

Telephone number

Obstetrician
Name

Address

Telephone number

Family Physician
Name

Address

Telephone number

Nurse-Midwife
Name

Address

Telephone number

Childbirth Education Class Teacher
Name

Address

Telephone number

Car/taxi service
Name

Telephone number

Pharmacy
Name

Address

Telephone number

PLANNING TO CONCEIVE

Fundamental to trying to get pregnant is evaluating your lifestyle and that of your partner, and making adjustments to ensure that both of you are in the best possible health. Ideally, this should be done at least one month, but preferably three months, beforehand.

Eliminate alcohol and stop smoking
Alcohol, smoking, and caffeine can be harmful to an expectant woman, her fetus, and newborn, and women who plan on becoming pregnant should not drink alcohol (see page 14). It is vital that both partners stop smoking and cut down on caffeine intake when trying to conceive.

Adjust diet and weight
At least one month, and preferably three, prior to conception you should make certain you are eating a diet rich in essential nutrients (see page 9) and low in fatty or sugary foods. You should also supplement your diet with foods containing folate (see page 9). Being overweight can cause problems during pregnancy, while being underweight can affect your reproductive cycle (see page 8) and chances of conception. Check with your doctor to see if your weight needs adjusting. Generally, it's not a good idea to go on a crash diet during pregnancy, because your unborn baby may suffer from a lack of nutrients essential for his development.

Work on your emotional well-being
Pregnancy, birth, and parenthood will deeply and irrevocably affect your relationships, especially that with your partner. Most parents are overwhelmed by the joys and challenges a new baby presents, though some may suffer from anxiety, resentment, and even depression. Use the time before conception to talk with your partner and discuss any doubts or insecurities.

Adjust your contraception
If you are using the contraceptive pill or an IUD (coil), switch to the diaphragm, cap, or condoms about three months before you plan to conceive. This will ensure you have at least one normal menstrual cycle before you become pregnant. If you conceive while you are still using the pill or an IUD, talk to your healthcare provider.

Seek genetic counseling
If there is a history of hereditary diseases, such as hemophilia or cystic fibrosis in your family, or if you know that you and your partner have incompatible blood types (see page 22), consider seeing a genetic counselor for advice before you conceive. Depending on ethnic background, other tests may be offered.

Get into shape
Your body will undergo many changes during pregnancy, so use the time before you conceive to attain a certain level of physical fitness (see page 29). Being physically fit will also help you have an easier delivery.

Mom-to-be

Ideally, you should be in the best possible shape for conception and future parenthood, having stopped smoking, stopped drinking alcohol, cut down on caffeine, and avoided unnecessary medications. You also should have moved away from, or be planning to leave, any potentially hazardous work situation (see page 44). If you or anyone in your immediate family suffers from a preexisting disease, discuss with your doctor any possible risks this may pose to a pregnancy.

BASAL BODY TEMPERATURE CHART

Dates covered: Month _____ Day _____ Year _____ to Month _____ Day _____ Year _____

Cycle Day	1	2	3	4	5	6	7	8	9	10	11	12	13	14	15	16	17	18	19	20	21	22	23	24	25	26	27	28
Weekday																												
Date																												
Time																												
99.0°F																												
98.9°F																												
98.8°F																												
98.6°F																												
98.5°F																												
98.3°F																												
98.0°F																												
97.9°F																												
97.7°F																												
97.5°F																												
97.3°F																												
97.2°F																												
97.1°F																												
97°F																												

Either photocopy three copies of this chart or print up a similar one from the internet. Mark a dot next to your temperature on each day of the three months and join the dots. You will soon see two patterns of temperature emerging—lower and higher. You are more likely to conceive when your temperature is higher and it is then that you should have more frequent intercourse.

Basal body temperature

Your basal body temperature can be measured on a digital basal body thermometer and charted to detect rises in temperature—the most likely time of ovulation. Now your temperature should hover near the 97.9°F mark but, hopefully, this will rise next week.

Record your change in body temperature by taking a reading each morning, before you get out of bed.

DATES FOR YOUR DIARY

MONDAY	TUESDAY	WEDNESDAY	THURSDAY	FRIDAY	SATURDAY/SUNDAY

FERTILIZATION

During your reproductive life, your uterus prepares for pregnancy every month, in the form of your menstrual cycle. Day one of your cycle is the first day of menstrual bleeding, when the lining (endometrium) of your uterus is shed. When bleeding stops, the endometrium is rebuilt. At about day five an ovum, or egg, starts to mature inside a fluid-filled sac (the follicle) in one of the two ovaries situated close to your fallopian tubes. In a 28-day cycle, at about day 14 when the follicle is mature, it ruptures and releases the egg. The ruptured follicle becomes the corpus luteum. This structure makes the hormone progesterone, which plays a vital role in helping your body adapt to pregnancy and in the early development of the embryo, if fertilization occurs. If you are to conceive, during ejaculation millions of your partner's sperm travel from your vagina to the fallopian tube. A few hundred sperm will make it to a waiting egg and release an enzyme that will allow one of them to penetrate its protective coating. This is the moment of fertilization. Should one of your partner's sperm penetrate your egg, all other sperm are prevented from doing so.

CONCEIVING TWINS

There are two types of twins: identical and nonidentical (or fraternal). Identical twins develop from the fertilization of a single egg by a single sperm. The egg divides into a zygote (two cells) then separates into two zygotes. These zygotes continue dividing in the normal way to eventually produce two fetuses with identical genes. Identical twins may or may not share a placenta and amniotic sac, but each twin has his own umbilical cord. Nonidentical twins develop when two eggs are fertilized by two separate sperm. Each fetus has his own placenta and individual genetic make-up.

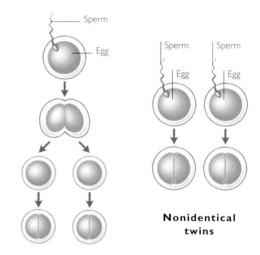

Identical twins

Nonidentical twins

Sperm meet egg
The tiny sperm are dwarfed by the ovum; here they attempt to pierce the zona pellucida, the ovum's protective covering.

Mom-to-be

Ovulation usually occurs 14 days prior to your next period, so, if you have a 28-day cycle, day 14 is when you are most likely to conceive. On this, or any adjusted date (due to the length of your cycle), you should start having regular sex with your partner. The body of this "lucky" sperm dissolves and its nucleus, containing your partner's genetic material, fuses with that of the egg, which contains yours.

Because ovulation usually occurs around day 14, a missed menstrual period two weeks later should indicate pregnancy. Traditionally, pregnancy is dated from the first day of your last menstrual period (LMP). However, if you are said to be four weeks pregnant (that is, it is four weeks after your LMP), your fetus' age and the period of gestation is only two weeks.

Baby

The sex of your baby is determined by two of the 46 chromosomes that make up his or her genetic blueprint. The egg and sperm each carry one. The egg has an X chromosome but the sperm has either an X or a Y chromosome. If an X-bearing sperm fertilizes the egg, you will have a girl; if the sperm carries a Y chromosome, you will have a boy. Therefore, the father determines his baby's gender.

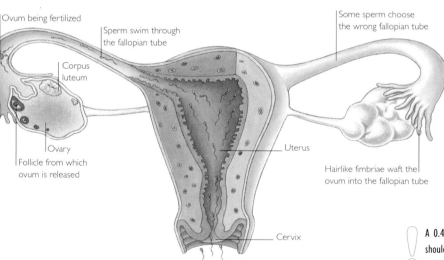

Ovum being fertilized

Sperm swim through the fallopian tube

Corpus luteum

Ovary

Follicle from which ovum is released

Some sperm choose the wrong fallopian tube

Uterus

Hairlike fimbriae waft the ovum into the fallopian tube

Cervix

Fertilization

This usually takes place in one of the fallopian tubes. Although as many as 300 million sperm are ejaculated into the vagina, only a few hundred reach the tube, and only one will fertilize the egg.

A 0.4°F rise in temperature this week should indicate ovulation. Confirm with an ovulation predictor kit.

DATES FOR YOUR DIARY

MONDAY	TUESDAY	WEDNESDAY	THURSDAY	FRIDAY	SATURDAY/SUNDAY

HEALTHY EATING

Your baby receives all her nourishment via your bloodstream, so it's important that you maintain a healthy diet. Any extra calories—approximately 300 per day (if you are underweight)—would only be necessary in the last three months when your baby is putting on fat. The need for protein, which is vital for creating new tissue, more than doubles during pregnancy, as does the requirement for calcium, needed for the baby's bone and teeth formation—at least in the last three months.

Iron is essential for the formation of hemoglobin, the oxygen-carrying pigment in red blood cells, and your baby's increasing volume of blood relies on a healthy supply of iron from your diet. Lack of iron—as well as vitamin B_{12} and folic acid, which aid the development of healthy blood cells—may result in anemia.

Folate (folic acid) is vital for preventing spina bifida, a neural tube disorder, so you should take a supplement containing 400 mcg folic acid starting three months prior to conception. Talk to your doctor about prenatal vitamin supplements and continued consumption of folate to ensure you are getting all the important nutrients you need. Some prescribed medications reduce your body's ability to absorb folate, so make sure you check with your doctor, who may prescribe a higher dose of folate.

Fluid intake

To keep your skin looking good and to maintain a healthy circulation and digestion, it's also important to drink at least eight 8-ounce glasses of fluids—preferably water—a day. During pregnancy, the volume of blood flowing around your body doubles so you need to maintain a high fluid intake.

SOURCES OF ESSENTIAL NUTRIENTS

Vitamin A	Dairy products, eggs, oily fish, yellow, orange, and green vegetables
Vitamin B_1	Whole grains, brewer's yeast, nuts, legumes, green leafy vegetables, pork
Vitamin B_2	Whole grains, green vegetables, eggs
Vitamin B_3	Whole grains, brewer's yeast, oily fish, eggs, milk
Vitamin B_5	Eggs, legumes, nuts, whole grains, avocados
Vitamin B_6	Eggs, salmon, peanuts, bananas, soybeans, sunflower seeds.
Vitamin B_{12}	Eggs, meat, oysters, milk
Folate	Leafy green vegetables, oranges, legumes
Vitamin C	Citrus fruits, strawberries, bell peppers, tomatoes, kiwi, mangoes, blueberries
Vitamin D	Fortified milk, oily fish (canned sardines), margarine, egg yolk, sunlight
Vitamin E	Oily fish, green leafy vegetables, broccoli, nuts, egg yolk, whole grains, unrefined oils
Calcium	Dairy products, canned sardines and salmon including bones, leafy green vegetables, legumes
Iron	Red meat, legumes, eggs, leafy green vegetables
Zinc	Vegetables, eggs, whole grains, nuts, sunflower seeds, watermelon and dried fruit, onions, beets, peas and legumes.

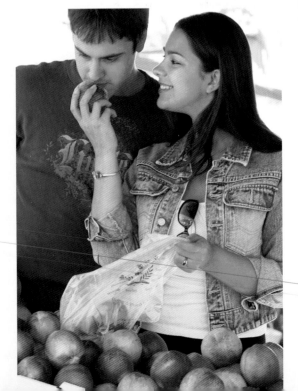

Snacking

Avoid fatty, sugary foods like cookies and pastries. Instead, choose fresh fruit and vegetables. Fruit is generally refreshing and contains fiber, which helps prevent constipation, a common complaint in pregnancy (see page 46).

Mom-to-be

Roughly seven days after fertilization, the morula—a solid ball of cells—implants in the lining of your uterus (the endometrium). As the ball of cells matures it becomes a blastocyst, secreting substances that trigger profound changes in your body, including the halting of the menstrual cycle.

Baby

After an egg has been fertilized, conception has been achieved, and cells begin to multiply at a tremendous rate. In just seven days, a single cell transforms into a ball of hundreds. Even though you can't discern much organization—even under a microscope—the cells are already grouping in a predetermined way. Some are destined to become the embryo, others to form the support structures (villi and placenta) that will nurture it. How this happens is still largely a mystery, but we do know that it involves a complex series of interactions.

The blastocyst, a hollow, fluid-filled ball of cells, burrows into the top part of the uterus. This happens between days four and seven, though it may not be firmly implanted until day ten. Cells from the outer coating of the blastocyst project rootlike attachments, called villi, into the endometrium. Villi allow an exchange of nutrients and waste between your bloodstream and the developing embryo. This connection will eventually mature into the placenta, the organ that will feed and protect your growing baby in the months ahead. Meanwhile, the lining of the uterus grows over the blastocyst, sealing it in.

From egg to embryo

The fertilized egg divides within hours to give a two-cell zygote, which continues to divide and subdivide until it forms a solid ball the size of a pinhead, the morula. After about four days, the morula transforms itself into a fluid-filled ball of approximately 100 cells, the blastocyst, from which the placenta and embryo will develop.

Making love every two days this week (and the last) will increase your chances of conceiving.

DATES FOR YOUR DIARY

MONDAY	TUESDAY	WEDNESDAY	THURSDAY	FRIDAY	SATURDAY/SUNDAY

MENU PLANNING

Eating well does not mean worrying about calorie consumption. In fact, it means being aware of the quality and nutritional content of the foods you eat. Certain nutrients are essential for a healthy pregnancy (see page 10), and as long as you make sure you have the recommended daily intake of these, your body should be able to adjust to the demands of a pregnancy very easily.

It is important to eat a wide variety of foods during pregnancy, because foods supply different nutrients in varying quantities. Citrus fruits, for example, provide vitamin C, which aids iron absorption and cell function, and sardines contain vitamin D, vital for sustaining the immune system.

Eating small meals frequently throughout the day will help you digest your food more effectively and give you more consistent energy. Eating small meals may also be helpful if you suffer from morning sickness.

Below is a suggested menu for one day (annotated to show what nutrients the foods provide). This is only a guide, so try to vary it with similar alternatives to suit your own preferences.

FOODS TO AVOID

- High-fat foods; sugary foods. These lack nutrients.
- Unpasteurized milk, juices, and apple cider, soft, unpasteurized cheeses (often labeled "fresh"), such as feta, goat, Brie, Camembert, and blue-veined cheeses, packaged salads, cooked food chilled for reheating, and pâtés. These have all been found to contain listeria, a bacteria that in rare cases can cause miscarriage or stillbirth.
- Raw or undercooked meats and poultry. These may cause toxoplasmosis, a disease that can bring about fetal brain damage and blindness. Processed meats like wieners and deli meats must be well cooked.
- Raw and undercooked eggs, and foods containing raw eggs, including mayonnaise, mousse, and tiramisù. They may contain salmonella bacteria, which can cause severe vomiting and diarrhea.
- Liver. Too much vitamin A can be harmful in pregnancy.
- Fish that are high in mercury, including shark, swordfish, king mackerel, or tilefish.

DAILY MENU

Breakfast
Eggs and wholewheat bread
(B and E vitamins, fiber, iron)
Yogurt flavored with fruits
(calcium, vitamin C, fiber)
A small glass of orange juice
(vitamin C and fluids)

Morning snack
Wholewheat bread (fiber) with peanut butter (protein, fiber, vitamin E, folic acid)
Bananas (potassium)
A glass of milk (protein, calcium)

Lunch
Broccoli and cheese soup
(folic acid, calcium, protein)
Sardines (calcium, vitamin D)
Potatoes (vitamin C, fiber, carbohydrates)

Afternoon snack
Sticks of raw vegetables, such as carrots and celery (vitamins, minerals)
Wholewheat crackers (fiber, carbohydrates)

Evening snack
Cheese and crackers (calcium and fiber)
A glass of milk (protein, calcium)

Dinner
Chicken (protein)
Whole-grain rice (carbohydrates, fiber)
Vegetables (vitamins, minerals)
Fresh fruit (fiber, vitamins, natural sugars)

Mom-to-be

If you suspect you may be pregnant, only a blood test will give you the most accurate result at this stage because home pregnancy tests are unable to detect the very small quantities of the pregnancy hormone, human chorionic gonadotropin (hCG), which the placenta has now secreted into your blood. While you wait to see whether or not your period arrives, you may experience a few pregnancy symptoms similar to premenstrual ones, such as queasiness or heavy breasts.

Baby

The blastocyst arrives in the uterus. Comprising hundreds of cells, it begins to attach itself to the uterine wall. The cells grow into the chorionic villi, which will later become the placenta. Released enzymes then pierce the uterine lining, causing tissue breakdown and providing nourishing blood cells on which the chorionic villi feed. The implantation process takes about 13 days.

Once the blastocyst implants, its cells begin to separate into layers. The top layer becomes the embryo and amniotic cavity and the lower layer becomes the yolk sac. The yolk sac will manufacture blood cells for the embryo until its own bone marrow is ready to take over the job (see page 65). The embryo further divides into three layers, as below.

Development of the embryo

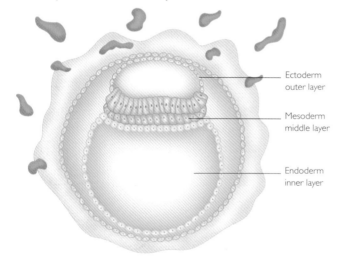

Ectoderm
outer layer

Mesoderm
middle layer

Endoderm
inner layer

Cell sandwich

Here you see the embryonic cell layers. The inner layer develops into the lungs, liver, bladder, thyroid gland, gastrointestinal system, and pancreas; the middle layer forms the skeleton, muscles, heart, circulation, and kidneys; the outer layer will become the brain and nervous system, teeth, and skin.

You may want to try a home pregnancy test to see if you have conceived.

DATES FOR YOUR DIARY

MONDAY	TUESDAY	WEDNESDAY	THURSDAY	FRIDAY	SATURDAY/SUNDAY

POTENTIAL HAZARDS

Smoking

Stop smoking and avoid smoke-filled environments. Smoking inhalation can result in preterm delivery, miscarriage, placenta previa, placental abruption, and preterm rupture of the membranes. After birth, it may also lead to Sudden Infant Death Syndrome (SIDS). If your partner or any other household member smokes, it will affect your baby's health leading to respiratory problems and even SIDS. Even passive smoking (being in a smoke-filled room) is very dangerous, because it could result in low birth weight and developmental disorders. The use of nicotine substitutes or antismoking medications is not recommended while pregnant.

Foodborne infections

Certain foods (see page 12), as well as preparation techinques, can result in harmful organisms damaging your unborn baby, as well as giving you food poisoning. Wash your hands and all equipment thoroughly before and after cooking, use separate cutting boards for meats, and make sure food is refrigerated properly. Do not handle cat litter boxes.

Household cleaning products

Cleaning products used in the home, and even some personal care products, can contain chemicals that are dangerous to a developing fetus. Avoid contact with pesticides and highly toxic products, such as oven cleaner, and always ventilate rooms well while cleaning.

Alcohol

The Office of the Surgeon General states that there is no known safe amount of alcohol use during pregnancy or while trying to get pregnant and advises women who are pregnant or who plan on becoming pregnant not to drink alcohol. All types of alcohol are equally harmful, including all wines and beer. Several conditions, including Fetal Alcohol Spectrum Disorders have been linked to alcohol consumption. A woman should not drink alcohol if she is sexually active and does not use effective contraception to avoid exposing her baby to alcohol before she knows she is pregnant. Nearly half of all pregnancies in the US are unplanned; most women will not know they are pregnant for up to 4 to 6 weeks.

Caffeine

Too much caffeine reduces the absorption of nutrients and can result in low birth weight or miscarriage. In addition to tea and coffee, caffeine is found also in colas, energy drinks, and chocolate, as well as in cold-and-flu remedies and some painkillers. Limit your intake to less than 200 mg a day (1 to 2 small coffees a day).

Medications and drugs

Few medicines have been established as safe to use while pregnant, so always discuss the pros and cons with your healthcare provider if you are prescribed medication, including nonprescription painkillers. If you are already on medication for a chronic condition or illness, such as diabetes or high blood pressure, make sure you dicuss the medication with your doctor in case a change in treatment is required, or the dosage needs to be adjusted. For short-term illnesses like colds, ask the pharmacist what treatment is best, since most over-the-counter medicine isn't advisable when pregnant.

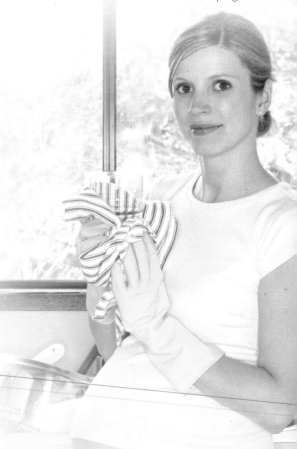

Mom-to-be

A home pregnancy test now may be able to confirm that you are pregnant, which you should suspect after missing a period. If test results are negative, you may want to repeat the test a few days later, particularly if your period has still not arrived. If the test is positive, think about whether you tell people now or wait until after the first trimester (after week 12), when complications are less likely.

Your breasts may be feeling fuller and more tender and you may suffer from fatigue. If you start to feel a little nauseous—particularly in the morning—try eating smaller meals and milder-tasting foods to see if that will settle your stomach. Of course, you may not be feeling any different. However, if you are, and these symptoms then disappear, you may want to seek advice from your healthcare provider. This may be a sign of a pregnancy complication.

Make sure you pay attention to risks. Never drink alcohol or smoke, and avoid exposure to second-hand smoke, or fumes from cleaning products (see page 14).

Baby

Shaped almost like a dumbbell, the embryo, at a gestational age of three weeks, has a groove down her back which seals up to form the neural tube. On both sides of this tube, specialized tissues known as somites arise, which will become muscle and other structures. A bulge is beginning to develop where your baby's heart will be and rudimentary blood vessels are growing into place. At this stage the yolk sac (rather than the placenta) provides nutrients and produces blood and sex cells.

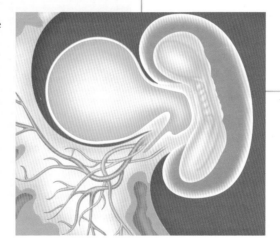

Support structures

As the primitive embryo floats within her amniotic sac, her umbilical cord is attaching to the placenta (lower left) so that nutrients must be supplied by her yolk sac (center).

Make an appointment this week to visit your healthcare provider to confirm your pregnancy, if you like. If you are pregnant, you can book your first prenatal appointment.

DATES FOR YOUR DIARY

MONDAY	TUESDAY	WEDNESDAY	THURSDAY	FRIDAY	SATURDAY/SUNDAY

FINDING OUT YOU'RE PREGNANT

Sometimes women know instinctively when they are pregnant. This may be due to the almost immediate surge in estrogen, prolonged high levels of progesterone, and the presence of the pregnancy hormone, human chorionic gonadotropin (hCG), which starts production about a week after conception. Most women, however, use a home pregnancy test. These check the levels of hCG (human chorionic gonadotropin) in your urine. Some tests ask you to hold a stick in your urine flow, others require that urine is passed first into a clean container and then a few drops squeezed from the dropper provided onto a window or an oblong stick. Usually, the result appears within minutes and can be read by looking for a colored line in a window on the stick. You should test the first urine you pass after you wake up in the morning, because this will contain the most hCG.

Early indications

The clearest sign that you may be pregnant is a missed period, although there are other reasons why menstruation may be delayed, such as stress, illness, extreme fluctuations in weight, or your body's adjustment to your coming off the pill, for example.

Tender, enlarged breasts can be a sign of pregnancy; it's not unusual for breast changes to begin a few days after conception.

You may also feel much more tired than usual. This may be due to the high levels of progesterone, a hormone that can have a sedative effect. Fatigue also can result

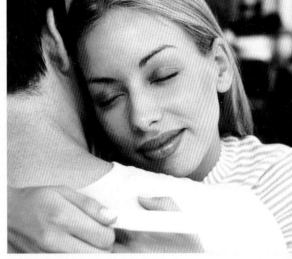

Performing a urine test
HCG can be detected in your urine four weeks after your last menstrual period. If you think you are pregnant—have missed your period—but the test is negative, you should try again a few days later.

from an increase in your metabolism, which is the body's way of coping with the strain on your vital organs and the support required for the growing embryo. This is why it is important to get plenty of rest.

Wanting to urinate frequently is another common sign as the enlarging uterus puts pressure on your bladder. After about 14 weeks, this will lessen as the uterus rises up into your abdomen.

Changes in taste and smell are normal, too. You may start to feel queasy when smelling or eating particular foods, develop an aversion to coffee, or start to crave a certain food. You may have a strange metallic taste in your mouth.

Your mood might change rapidly, making you overly emotional or weepy. This is caused by the action of the pregnancy hormones.

See page 18 for how to deal with fatigue and with nausea or morning sickness, a common early complaint.

EXPECTED DELIVERY DATE

The date of your baby's birth will be calculated 40 weeks from the first day of your last menstrual period (LMP). At 40 weeks of pregnancy, however, your fetus is actually only 38 weeks old (see page 8). Your baby's estimated date of delivery (EDD) is only an approximation, however, and you may go into labor any time between weeks 38 and 42. Fewer than 5 percent of babies arrive on their EDD, and women expecting their first baby often have overdue pregnancies.

Mom-to-be

You may visit your healthcare prodvider this week to confirm your pregnancy (with a blood test) and to get an estimated delivery date. You can calculate this date as 40 weeks from the first day of your last menstrual period (see page 8).

You may notice further changes to your breasts: your nipples may be more prominent and the areole surrounding them may have darkened, and bluish veins may be apparent just under the skin.

A pregnancy is divided into three time periods, known as trimesters. The first trimester is up to week 12, during which time there is rapid fetal development. This is also the time when you are most at risk of a miscarriage (see page 18). The second trimester spans weeks 13 to 27 and the third trimester is from weeks 28 to 40.

Baby

Though just a tube, his heart is starting to beat, and his neural tube is closing in preparation for the development of the spinal cord. His brain is growing to fill his head and pigment is filling the optical vesicles, shallow orbs on the sides of his head.

A rudimentary digestive tract begins to form, together with the abdominal and chest cavities. Arm and leg buds have also developed, though an obvious tail is still visible on his curved body. His primitive lungs, liver, pancreas, and thyroid gland are starting to develop, his nostrils are becoming distinct, and his neck and jaw are developing.

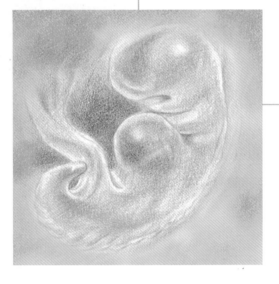

Taking shape

The embryo has a clear top and bottom, and is assuming a characteristic C-shape. His heart bulges and his developing spinal cord is clear.

BABY'S LENGTH AND WEIGHT
His length, from crown to rump, will be about the size of a lentil. The pregnancy sac is about ½ a teaspoon in volume.

If you haven't already seen your healthcare provider, contact them now to schedule your first prenatal visit.

DATES FOR YOUR DIARY

MONDAY	TUESDAY	WEDNESDAY	THURSDAY	FRIDAY	SATURDAY/SUNDAY

EARLY PREGNANCY COMPLAINTS

Some women sail through the first few weeks of pregnancy without any obvious symptoms. In fact, those who normally have irregular periods may not even realize they are pregnant for the first few months. Initially, the way you feel may be similar to how you felt just before your period started. For example, you may have suffered from heavy, sore breasts when you were premenstrual. However, nausea and fatigue tend to affect the majority of women to some degree.

Nausea

In the early weeks of pregnancy, the most common symptom is nausea, often accompanied by vomiting. Although commonly called morning sickness, it can strike at any time of the day. It occurs more often when you don't eat enough, so always keep some snacks, such as dry crackers or fresh fruit, handy. If you are affected

and you usually eat three standard meals a day, try changing your eating pattern to more frequent, smaller meals. Ginger root is good for combatting nausea. Use it fresh, adding it to cooking, drink it as a tea, take it as tablets in a health food supplement.

If you suffer from severe nausea, there are various medications that are safe to take and may be helpful. Seek advice from your healthcare provider.

Because pregnancy heightens your sense of smell, some familiar foods can set off nausea. Common examples are tea and coffee and foods that are high in fat or sugar. Other scents, including your favorite perfume, also may make you feel nauseated.

Tiredness

Most women are surprised at how exhausted they feel early on in pregnancy. Fatigue may be a side effect of the physical changes taking place, including the dramatic rise in hormone levels. You need to get as much rest as you can: go to bed early at night and do gentle exercise to help you relax. Avoid caffeine and sugary foods and concentrate on foods with a low glycemic index.

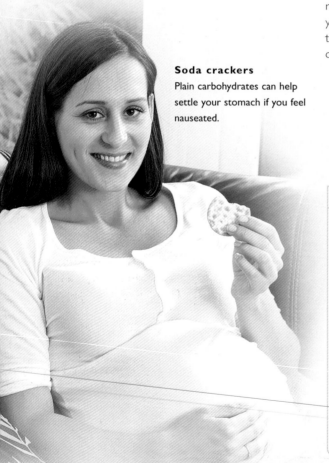

Soda crackers
Plain carbohydrates can help settle your stomach if you feel nauseated.

PAIN AND BLEEDING

These are not normal symptoms and may indicate a miscarriage or ectopic pregnancy, both of which are medical emergencies.

- It is estimated that 20 to 40 percent of all pregnancies end in miscarriage, most in the first three months. Symptoms include heavy, clotted bleeding, and cramps.
- An ectopic pregnancy occurs when the embryo implants itself outside the uterus, usually in the fallopian tubes. Symptoms include abdominal pain on one side, vaginal bleeding, nausea, shoulder pain, and dizziness.

Mom-to-be

Breast discomfort—tingling and heaviness—may be apparent; this is caused by stimulation of the milk-producing glands.

You may also feel irritable, and you'll almost certainly start to feel more tired than previously without extra exertion. This is due to your raised levels of progesterone. Even at this early stage you need to make time for relaxation (see page 34).

You may start having to urinate more frequently and may notice an excess of saliva, an increased vaginal discharge, and some unexpected nasal congestion.

Internal changes are also happening—your heart rate rises steeply and your metabolic rate starts to increase—but you may be unaware of these.

Baby

Facial features begin to appear: eyes are pigmented disks on each side of the head; nostrils little openings; the mouth an indentation. Ears are developing on the sides of her neck. Her bumpy head is much bigger than the rest of her body. Arm and leg buds are protruding more and elbows and shoulders are discernible, as are paddle-shaped hands and feet. Her brain has divided into segments and her heart beats at about 150 beats per minute (twice as fast as yours). Muscle fibers are growing in preparation for movement, and her tail is disappearing.

In the lungs, air passageways (bronchi) are forming and the intestines are developing, part of which bulge into the umbilical cord. Her internal sex organs are nearly complete. The umbilical cord is also growing as the placenta matures.

Budding genius
Limb buds and the brain are developing fast. Your baby's head contains some distinguishing features, such as the eyes. Inside, primitive organs continue to grow, including the liver and lungs.

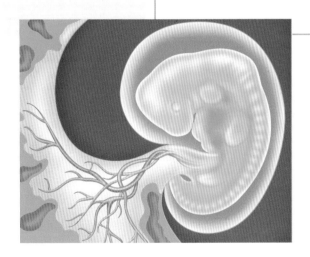

BABY'S LENGTH
From crown to rump, she will be about as big as a blueberry.

Stock up on supplies of fresh ginger, soda crackers, and other bland, easy-to-digest carbohydrates to relieve morning sickness.

DATES FOR YOUR DIARY

MONDAY	TUESDAY	WEDNESDAY	THURSDAY	FRIDAY	SATURDAY/SUNDAY

PRENATAL CARE

You should have checkups regularly throughout your pregnancy, though the number of visits to a healthcare provider and the timing of prenatal tests can vary depending on your insurance coverage and personal circumstances. The chart to the right sets out the range of suitable appointment dates and indicates possible procedures. If you are expecting twins or have a medical problem, you should be seen more often.

Your booking appointment

This first official prenatal visit to your doctor or health clinic will usually take longer and be more detailed than subsequent visits. You will be asked about your medical background, lifestyle, and family history of things such as multiple births and genetic disorders.

The health of your breasts, heart, and lungs will be checked, your abdomen palpated, your cervix examined; your weight and height may be measured. You will have a number of tests (see page 22) and you may be prescribed prenatal vitamins.

Subsequent visits

You and your unborn baby's progress will be monitored. Your caregiver will probably discuss diet and exercise with you, and you should take the opportunity to discuss any problems that may have arisen.

Try not to miss a prenatal appointment—it is vital that your pregnancy is monitored to ensure a healthy baby and safe birth.

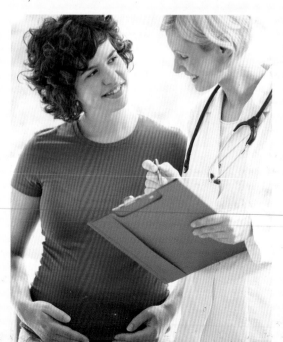

APPOINTMENTS FOR YOUR DIARY

FIRST TRIMESTER
Weeks 8 to 12
- First official prenatal appointment scheduled
- Blood testing for genetic conditions may be performed
- Due date estimated

Weeks 11 & 12
- Early/dating scan and fetal nuchal translucency test possible
- Chorionic villus sampling (CVS) possible
- Screening test possible

SECOND TRIMESTER
Weeks 13 to 15
- Early/dating scan and nuchal translucency test possible
- Chorionic villus sampling (CVS) possible
- Screening test possible

Week 16
- Prenatal appointment
- Blood test for Down syndrome may be offered
- Anomaly scan possible
- Amniocentesis possible
- Serum screening including alpha-fetoprotein (AFP) test possible

Week 17
- Serum screening including alpha-fetoprotein (AFP) test possible
- Amniocentesis possible

Week 18
- Serum screening including alpha-fetoprotein (AFP) test possible
- Anomaly scan possible
- Amniocentesis possible

Weeks 20 to 23
- Prenatal appointment
- Serum screening including alpha-fetoprotein (AFP) test possible
- Anomaly scan possible
- Fetal blood sampling possible

Week 24
- Prenatal appointment
- Fetal blood sampling possible

Weeks 26 & 27
- Glucose screen possible
- Fetal blood sampling possible

THIRD TRIMESTER
Weeks 28, 30, 32 & 34
- Prenatal appointment
- Blood test for anemia and/or glucose screen may be offered
- Fetal blood sampling possible

Week 36
- Prenatal appointment
- Test for Group B Strep may be offered
- Fetal blood sampling possible

Weeks 37 to 40
- Prenatal appointment
- Baby's size and position assessed
- Fetal blood sampling possible

Your prenatal visits

Raise any concerns about your pregnancy at your checkups; it is a good idea to make a list of things you want to discuss beforehand.

Mom-to-be

Although your uterus is starting to swell it probably won't show just yet. Generally, the only people who will notice at this stage are your healthcare provider—who can feel the enlargement when doing a pelvic exam—and you; your clothes may feel tighter around your waistline. While nausea, tiredness, and mood swings are common symptoms at this time and may occasionally prove unpleasant, view them as signs that your body is adapting itself to the demands of pregnancy and the needs of your growing baby.

Baby

His body is unfurling slightly as the spine straightens and his trunk gets longer. His head, bent forward on his chest, is much bigger than his body, and his facial features continue to develop. His arms and legs have become longer and project forward. At the tips, tiny fingers and toes are growing.

He has a rudimentary nose and tongue and his upper lip is forming. His eyes, with discernible eyelids, are open and spaced far apart, and his inner ears are forming. His heart, brain, liver, lungs, and kidneys are now present in a basic form, and his intestines are so long that they are developing outside the abdomen, in a sac adjacent to the umbilical cord.

Head strong

A feature of both a developing fetus and a newborn is that the head is his largest part. Your baby has started to move around, thanks to the firming up and lengthening of leg and arm tissue and the development of his joints.

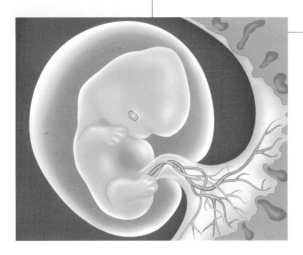

BABY'S LENGTH AND WEIGHT
His length, from crown to rump, will be around the same as a kidney bean and his weight is about 0.1 ounce.

If your first official prenatal appointment takes place this week, be sure to allow plenty of time for it.

DATES FOR YOUR DIARY

MONDAY	TUESDAY	WEDNESDAY	THURSDAY	FRIDAY	SATURDAY/SUNDAY

ROUTINE TESTS

Throughout your pregnancy your healthcare giver will perform a number of tests. These include regular checks of your blood pressure and any swelling in your hands and feet and measurements of your fundal height (the distance from the top of your uterus to your pelvic bone). The latter monitors the baby's size. Generally, you will only be weighed if you were over- or underweight when you started your pregnancy or if you don't seem to be gaining weight at a reasonable rate.

After week 16 your baby's heartbeat will also be monitored. Depending on your progress, other tests may also be performed (see chart page 20).

Blood tests

A blood test can usually confirm a pregnancy before a urine test. Once you are pregnant, a sample of your blood will be used to assess: your blood type; whether you have healthy glucose, iron, and hemoglobin levels; whether you are immune to rubella; whether you have the hepatitis B virus, syphilus or HIV, or if you have a toxoplasmosis infection. Your blood also will be tested to see whether you are rhesus (Rh) positive or negative. This last result is very important, because if your baby is rhesus positive and you are rhesus negative, you can form antibodies to your baby's red blood cells, which will have serious consequences for your next rhesus-positive baby. Luckily, effective treatment is available for mother and baby.

Blood can also be used to check alpha-fetoprotein levels, which can indicate a risk of certain pregnancy complications (see page 36), including fetal abnormalities.

Urine tests

You will have to supply a urine sample at every prenatal appointment, which will be tested for protein. The presence of protein in your urine could indicate an infection or, more seriously, preeclampsia (see page 58). Your urine will also be tested for the presence of glucose, which may indicate gestational diabetes, a type of diabetes unique to pregnancy, in which the body fails to produce enough insulin to cope with the increased blood sugar levels.

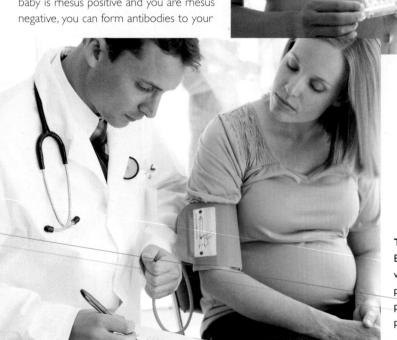

Testing blood pressure
Blood pressure is monitored at every visit. An elevated reading may indicate pregnancy-induced hypertension or preeclampsia. An average reading during pregnancy is about 120/70.

Mom-to-be

Your body shape will not yet reveal that you are pregnant. The pregnancy hormone hCG (human chorionic gonadotropin) is now at its peak, however, and you will notice certain changes, such as your facial skin becoming smoother and plumper, although there may be an outbreak of pimples. You may find that you need to wash your hair less frequently because it tends to become less oily. Also, your breasts may be fuller or feel slightly tender. At times you may notice some vaginal discharge in varying amounts. This is natural, and usually not a cause for concern. If, however, your discharge is very thick and there is itching or a strange odor, let your doctor know, because it may be a mild vaginal infection.

Baby

The embryo looks more like a baby now. Her head is large, her tail has disappeared, and her back is straighter; her nose and jaw are complete, and her neck is more apparent. A protective membranous lid covers her eyes. Her skin is thickening and hair follicles are developing.

By now her fingers are almost complete and separate, her arms and legs are elongating, and she has knee and elbow joints. Her ribcage is closing to protect her heart and her intestines are starting to move their way back into the abdominal cavity, which is now big enough to house them.

Making a move
Although you can't feel anything, your baby is now able to move both her arms (which contain hands and fingers) and her legs (which contain feet and toes).

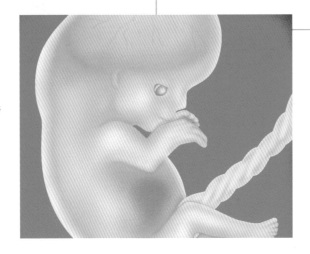

BABY'S LENGTH AND WEIGHT
Her length, from crown to rump, will be approximately 1 inch, and she will weigh about 0.14 ounce.

Purchase a properly fitting cotton maternity bra to support tender breasts.

DATES FOR YOUR DIARY

MONDAY	TUESDAY	WEDNESDAY	THURSDAY	FRIDAY	SATURDAY/SUNDAY

BIRTH CHOICES

There is a wide range of childbirth options, including where to deliver and types of pain relief (see page 74). While it is a woman's right to decide how she wants to give birth, a certain type of delivery may be advised for medical reasons, for example, if you are expecting twins or your baby is in a side-lying or breech position. Most women will decide based on their health histories, personal preferences, and financial ability.

Hospital birth

If you have chosen an obstetrician or family practitioner as your healthcare provider, you will most likely be making plans to give birth in a hospital. However, the number of births attended by nurse-midwives in hospital settings is increasing. Some families feel more comfortable having access to technology in case complications arise. In a hospital, though, there may be more restrictions during labor and birth. Be sure to take a tour of your chosen hospital before giving birth and familiarize yourself with all the guidelines and policies regarding laboring techniques, routine interventions, use of cameras or video, and newborn care.

Birth centers

For women with a low-risk pregnancy seeking a more natural birth experience, a birth center might be the solution. It is always best to research the birthing centers in your location to find one that best meets your needs. You can expect to be looked after by a team including nurse-midwives, direct-entry midwives (if they are legal in your state; see page 60), or nurses working with an obstetrician. Some facilities are free-standing while others are on hospital grounds or within a hospital. If you are considering a home birth, or if you and your partner want to compromise on a birth location, a birthing center can be a good option.

Home birth

When giving birth at home, nurse-midwives are the main carers. Many women who want to avoid any interventions and seek a family-centered experience tend to choose home birth, but this is recommended only for low-risk pregnancies. At home, women can have as much time as they need to give birth naturally without drugs and medical interventions, and have the most control over labor and birth, though they must remain open to the possible need to be taken to a hospital in the event of an unexpected complication. Throughout your pregnancy, the nurse-midwife will see you at home or in a clinic for prenatal checkups, and to ensure your pregnancy and birth are as risk-free as possible. See page 60 for more information on home births.

Natural childbirth

Available within many hospitals, birthing centers, and at all home deliveries, natural childbirth is one in which pain relief is achieved without drugs. Instead, a variety of noninvasive methods are used to ease the mother's pain. Many emphasize the "mind-body connection," unlike a medical birth. Such methods include controlled breathing; meditation; using labor aids; assuming different positions, such as kneeling, squatting, or rocking back and forth on a birthing ball; or the use of a birthing pool.

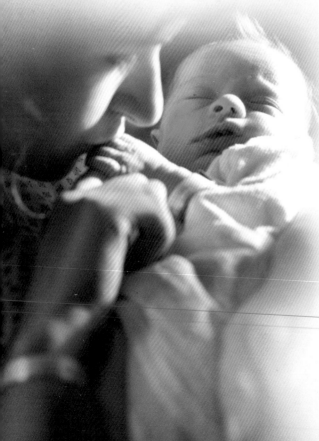

The birth of your choice

A homelike atmosphere, with dim lights, comfortable chairs, and cushions to arrange as you please will help you relax and gain more control over your delivery. Some hospitals and most birth centers have special, sympathetically furnished labor and delivery rooms.

Mom-to-be

High hormone levels will produce emotional as well as physical effects. It is perfectly natural to find yourself getting overwrought or having strange mood swings ranging from feelings of elation to weepiness.

Physical changes include the start of weight gain, potential softening of the gums, and a slightly swollen thyroid gland. Because your teeth are now more susceptible to bacteria and plaque, brush your teeth at least twice a day and floss regularly. Arrange to have a dental checkup, making sure you let the dentist know you are pregnant so X-rays can be avoided.

Now only two weeks from the end of your first trimester, you can look forward to a significant reduction in symptoms such as morning sickness.

Baby

Now known as a fetus (offspring or little one), his body is basically complete. His brain has grown large and his eyes and nose can be seen clearly. Eyelids have fused his eyes shut, which won't open now until week 27.

Twenty tooth buds for his deciduous teeth (also called milk teeth or baby teeth) are forming in his gums and taste buds on his tongue. Most of his joints, including wrists and ankles, are formed, and separated fingers and toes make him capable of a wide range of movements.

His nervous system is responsive and his fully developed heart beats at 140 beats per minute. His lungs, stomach, and intestines are still growing, while the kidneys move into their final position in the upper abdomen.

Hands, nose, fingers, knees, and toes

Most of these features are now present in miniature. Soon your baby will start to suck his thumb. Already he can make whole body movements, though only involuntary ones.

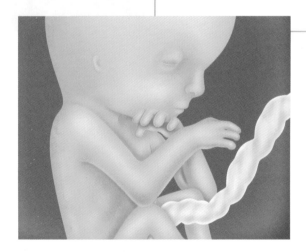

BABY'S LENGTH AND WEIGHT
His length, from crown to rump, will be around 1¼ to 1⅜ inches and he will weigh about 0.17 ounce.

You may be given an appointment for your first "dating" ultrasound this week (see page 26).

DATES FOR YOUR DIARY

MONDAY	TUESDAY	WEDNESDAY	THURSDAY	FRIDAY	SATURDAY/SUNDAY

EARLY SCREENING TESTS

To check that a pregnancy is healthy and a baby is developing normally, doctors use ultrasound scanning. Should problems be suspected, other, more invasive, tests are available.

Ultrasound

This involves transmitting short pulses of high frequency but low intensity sound waves through the uterus to produce an image of the developing baby and surrounding structures.

The first ultrasound may be performed as early as week 8 of pregnancy, although this varies up to about week 13 plus six days. The first ultrasound is often called the "dating" scan because it can reveal the age of the fetus, as well as whether a single baby or twins are present, and the location of the placenta. Later scans will show genitalia and therefore the baby's sex, the position she is lying in, and if there are any developmental abnormalities.

Scans performed in very early pregnancy are usually done transvaginally, using a special ultrasound probe inserted into the vagina. Later ultrasounds are usually performed transabdominally, using a transducer that is moved across the mother's abdomen. In the scanning room, you will be asked to lie on your back next to the machinery and expose your abdomen. The examiner will rub gel, which acts as a conductor of sound waves, onto your abdomen and will then move a transducer back and forth over the area. An image of your baby will appear on the screen next to you. Most clinics give you a printout of the image for you to keep. The whole process should not take more than 30 minutes.

Nuchal translucency

Ultrasound will be used to check a fluid-filled area behind your baby's neck, which can be used to diagnose the possibility of Down syndrome (see page 36). This space will be measured and a computer program will provide an individualized risk assessment based on your age and the size of the fluid-filled area and in conjunction with certain blood tests. If there is a risk of Down syndrome or other abnormalities, chorionic villus sampling will be carried out.

Chorionic villus sampling (CVS)

A sample of placental tissue will be obtained by passing a catheter through the cervix or placing a needle through your abdomen. This will be analyzed to check for abnormalities of chromosome number or structure or certain specific genetic disorders. It is associated with a small risk of miscarriage. Ultrasound will be used to guide the doctor to the right location and to avoid injury to the baby.

An exciting moment
Ultrasound scanning gives you the opportunity to see your developing baby for the first time. Bone and other dense structures appear white on the screen and softer tissues, such as the heart and kidneys, gray. Ask the technician to point out the different body parts.

Mom-to-be

Your body is now burning up calories at a faster rate than it did before you were pregnant because your basal metabolic rate has risen by as much as 25 percent. The amount of blood being pumped around your body will also increase. This can make you feel much warmer than usual and you will probably perspire more, so drink plenty of fluids.

If you haven't had your first prenatal appointment yet, write down any questions you want to ask about your care and your baby's progress. Make sure you check up on your family's medical history because your healthcare provider will want to know about anything that could affect your baby.

Baby

All of her vital organs—brain, lungs, liver, kidneys, and intestines—are formed and increasing in volume. Her inner ears will finish forming by the end of the week and her eyes, which have moved to the center of her face, are developing irises. From now until about week 20 she will grow more rapidly. The placenta's blood vessels increase in number to provide her with essential nutrients. Hair and nails are growing and amniotic fluid begins to accumulate as the kidneys start to function. In her abdomen, the intestines are developing. Part of them still projects into the umbilical cord ("physiological herniation") but they will return to the abdomen next week.

Out of proportion

Your baby's head accounts for half of her body length. This is because her brain gets a head-start during development. The rest of her body will catch up in later months. She can now suck, swallow, and yawn.

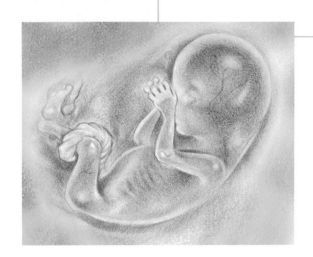

BABY'S LENGTH AND WEIGHT
Her length, from crown to rump, will be around 1¾ to 2⅓ inches and she will weigh about 0.28 ounce.

If your doctor recommends a CVS test, it will be performed around this week (see page 26).

DATES FOR YOUR DIARY

MONDAY	TUESDAY	WEDNESDAY	THURSDAY	FRIDAY	SATURDAY/SUNDAY

WEIGHT GAIN

The recommended weight gain for a healthy singleton pregnancy is about 20 to 30 pounds and 35 to 54 pounds for twins. If you are underweight, however, your doctor may suggest you gain more. If you are overweight, you may not need to gain much weight at all.

Piling on the pounds

At birth your baby will usually weigh less than 9 pounds. The rest of your weight gain during pregnancy, therefore, is made up of the placenta, the amniotic fluid, your increased blood volume, and enlarged uterus and breasts.

Pregnant women gain weight at different rates, so don't be alarmed if you get bigger sooner than your pregnant friends. During the first trimester (up to week 12), women tend to gain only 2 to 4 pounds. In the second trimester (weeks 13 to 27) they gain approximately

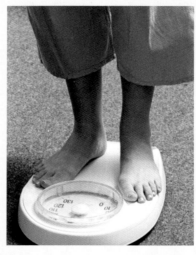

13 pounds, and during the final trimester (weeks 28 to 40), about 11 pounds. This is just an average, so, of course, your individual pattern of weight gain may differ. At week six there is usually little discernible difference in your

weight. You will notice an increase from about week 12, with the most rapid rise between weeks 20 and 30. After week 36, your weight will tend to remain about level. If you are prone to fluid retention toward the end of your pregnancy, there may be a further increase.

A sudden increase in weight may signify a condition known as preeclampsia, which can develop into eclampsia and both of these conditions can be life-threatening for the mother and the baby (see page 58). Luckily, however, due to the careful vigilance of prenatal health practitioners, preeclampsia is usually detected at an early stage and steps can be taken to reduce the chances of it becoming a serious danger.

Fluid retention

Some pregnant women experience fluid retention during their pregnancy, which will account for part of their weight gain. Fluid retention is most often due to dilation of the veins and pooling of blood. In rare cases, however, it may be associated with malfunctioning kidneys, heart and liver disorders, or poor circulation. Exercising frequently and wearing loose clothing can aid circulation. Wearing compression stockings (up to the groin) may also help.

Watching your weight

Try not to let your weight become an obsession. It is your body's duty to provide a nurturing environment for your growing baby and your increasing weight is a sign of this. In any case, much of the weight you put on during your pregnancy will be lost when your baby is born; breastfeeding (see page 68) can also be helpful for weight loss.

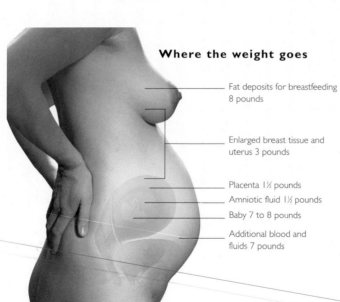

Where the weight goes

Fat deposits for breastfeeding 8 pounds

Enlarged breast tissue and uterus 3 pounds

Placenta 1½ pounds
Amniotic fluid 1½ pounds
Baby 7 to 8 pounds

Additional blood and fluids 7 pounds

Mom-to-be

Your uterus has grown to about 4 inches in width. It is now too big to sit in your pelvis and begins to move up into your abdomen, so if you've had to urinate frequently, this should now ease. Your doctor can predict more accurately your EDD (estimated date of delivery) from your baby's crown-to-rump height, which will be measured on an ultrasound scan.

Although you won't be aware of it, your heart may start to speed up by a few beats per minute, in order to cope with the increased volume of blood circulating in your body.

Any morning sickness should have disappeared, or will do soon. You may have your first prenatal appointment this week or some tests; be prepared!

Your baby

Fetal growth continues rapidly—he has doubled in size in the last three weeks, his face looks more human, and his organs continue to grow. He is growing hair and nails, and his bones are hardening as calcium is laid down. He is much less at risk of developing congenital abnormalities now.

The pituitary gland, at the base of the brain, is beginning to produce hormones. His vocal chords are starting to form. His digestive system is able to contract to push food through his bowels and he can absorb glucose. Genital organs have begun to form, but only an expert can confirm your baby's sex.

Floating free

Your baby makes the most of his buoyant environment by exercising his arms and legs with a range of fluid and supple movements. He is also capable of a range of facial expressions.

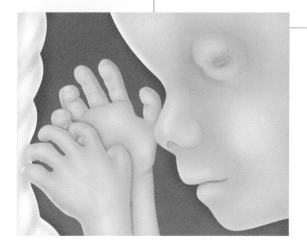

BABY'S LENGTH AND WEIGHT
His length, from crown to rump, will be around 2½ inches and he will weigh about 0.31 to 0.45 ounce.

If you have your prenatal appointment this week, ask whether you can stop taking your folic acid supplement.

DATES FOR YOUR DIARY

MONDAY	TUESDAY	WEDNESDAY	THURSDAY	FRIDAY	SATURDAY/SUNDAY

STAYING PHYSICALLY FIT

Exercise strengthens muscles, improves circulation, aids digestion, and increases stamina, so regular exercise during pregnancy will help combat common pregnancy complaints such as constipation, leg cramps, and tiredness. It also helps you adjust to the inevitable weight gain and prepares your body to cope with the major physical demands of labor. In addition, it releases chemical hormones called endorphins into your bloodstream, which invoke feelings of happiness and relaxation. These endorphins pass across the placenta, so your baby will also feel their positive effects.

Keeping fit throughout pregnancy will increase the likelihood of an easy labor and make regaining your pre-pregnancy fitness levels and shape much easier.

Suggested activities

Gentle swimming and walking are ideal for pregnancy, especially if you were not very active beforehand. Walking increases your circulation and aids digestion, while swimming tones your muscles and increases stamina. Neither of these is likely to put pressure on your joints, made vulnerable during pregnancy (see page 32).

Pelvic tilt

This will strengthen the muscles in the small of your back and help prevent backaches. Kneel on all fours with your back straight. Tuck in your pelvis by clenching your buttock muscles and arch your back. Hold for a few seconds, then release.

Prenatal pilates is the perfect pregnancy exercise: it helps improve posture and increases core strength, boosts circulation, and helps with fluid retention. Gentle exercises work muscles without straining joints, while the breathing exercises taught in pilates are beneficial in labor and for general relaxation.

Prenatal yoga offers the same physical benefits as pilates, but also aims at improving mental well-being and reducing stress through various levels of meditation.

Taking care

Be extra careful when weightlifting during pregnancy and avoid any heavy weights; weight training puts pressure on joints and ligaments, which are vulnerable during pregnancy, so consult with your doctor or personal trainer.

Listen to your body and stop your exercise session if you feel dizzy, too hot, too tired, or are in any pain.

Most doctors are of the opinion that vigorous sports should not be undertaken in the first trimester because the risk of miscarriage is greatest then. Although you should seek your healthcare provider's advice first, if you played a sport such as tennis regularly before you were pregnant, then usually it should not be a problem to continue playing it during the first and second trimesters.

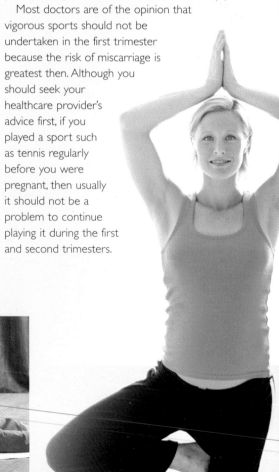

Mom-to-be

Now in your second trimester, the best period of your pregnancy may be beginning. You may well find your hunger increases or that you start to crave certain foods or find others unappetizing. You will probably start to feel more energetic since first trimester problems, such as nausea and fatigue, ease.

The placenta now produces hormones—mainly progesterone and estriol—previously produced by your ovaries; these play a vital role in maintaining your pregnancy and inducing the necessary bodily changes.

If you haven't already done so, you can announce your pregnancy now with confidence because the risk of complications is much less.

Baby

All her vital organs and structures are basically formed, but are still immature. Her intestines have moved farther into her body, her liver begins to excrete bile, and her pancreas starts to produce insulin. She is also moving constantly, though you can't feel the movements, and bone tissue is appearing. Her reflexes are improving as her nerve cells multiply and neurological development continues apace. If her palm encounters her umbilical cord, her fingers will curl around it.

Your baby has developed opposable thumbs—these are vital tools for all humans because they allow us to pick up, hold, and manipulate items.

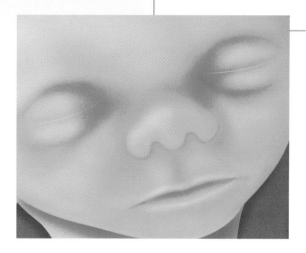

Front-facing features
Your baby's eyes are at the front of her face and her ears are nearing their final position. She can open and close her lips. Her neck supports her head movements.

BABY'S LENGTH AND WEIGHT
Her length, from crown to rump, will be around 3 inches and she will weigh about 0.7 ounce.

You'll probably have had your first trimester scan by now and will want to tell others about your pregnancy.

DATES FOR YOUR DIARY

MONDAY	TUESDAY	WEDNESDAY	THURSDAY	FRIDAY	SATURDAY/SUNDAY

POSTURE MATTERS

Many of the movements that we take for granted—standing, walking, and sitting—may need to be adjusted during pregnancy so that you preserve good posture. You need to carry your baby in your uterus in a way that is comfortable for both of you.

Good posture can help to alleviate any unnecessary strain on your back muscles. The hormone relaxin, released during pregnancy, results in softened and stretched ligaments, which can make your back vulnerable to strains. Moreover, as your abdomen enlarges and your baby becomes heavier, you may find yourself leaning backward or stooping forward to adjust your center of gravity. This can strain the muscles around your spine, resulting in a backache, particularly during the last trimester.

It's also a good idea to perform some stretches as part of your warm-up and cool-down during exercise sessions; keep your back straight and your body centrally weighted at all times.

Standing
Drop your shoulders so that they are relaxed. Tuck in your buttocks and straighten your back. Lengthen your neck and raise your head as though the center at the top is being pulled toward the ceiling. Avoid tensing your knees and keep your weight evenly spread between your toes and heels. When at the sink, work at waist height, using a large plastic dish tub on top of the sink if it is low. If ironing, lower the board and sit down to iron.

Sitting
Whether sitting in a chair or on the floor, always keep your back straight. When you sit in a chair, sit flush against the back of the chair so that it supports the small of your back. If your chair doesn't provide this support comfortably, you can place a small cushion or rolled-up towel in the small of your back. To prevent poor circulation, don't sit with your legs crossed and keep them raised whenever possible.

Lying down
Lie down slowly, and always from a sitting position. When you are seated, swing your legs slowly over the bed or couch so that they are parallel with your hips. Gently lower yourself onto your elbows, so they support the weight of your upper body. Using your hands, slide down into a lying position.

Getting up
Raise yourself from a prone (only in the first trimester) or supine position in a series of stages. First, roll onto your side. Next, raise yourself onto your elbows so they support your upper body, and push with your hands to ease yourself into a sitting position. Finally, keeping your back straight, slowly stand up from this position.

Lifting
Squat down next to the item, keeping your back straight. Bring the item close to you then lift it up using your leg and thigh muscles to support the weight.

Walking
For balanced posture, wear low-heeled shoes and walk with your feet parallel to each other.

Posture check

Look straight ahead and lengthen your neck, keeping your chin parallel to the floor

Relax your shoulders and open your chest

Tighten your abdominal muscles

Keep your pelvis tilted

Ensure that your knees are soft and in line with your ankles

Mom-to-be

At this stage of your pregnancy, your uterus is now swelling week by week. You can follow its progress by locating the top of the uterus—the fundus. The position of this will gradually move up your abdomen over the coming weeks. Lying flat on your back, position a measuring tape at "0 inches" on your pubic bone and count upward by ½ inch for every week of pregnancy. Your doctor, however, is more likely to monitor the growth of your uterus by using ultrasound than by fundal height measurements because it is more accurate.

If your doctor has advised a CVS (see page 25) or serum screening test, it may well take place this week.

Baby

Besides making smoother, more complex movements with his hands, and being able to squint and make various facial expressions, he can now "suck" his thumb. His nervous system is functioning and he "practices" breathing movements. It is easier now to determine his gender since his external genitalia are more developed.

This is also an important week for your baby's developing internal organs and his thyroid gland, which has matured and started to produce hormones. His kidneys are functioning well now, producing and releasing urine into the amniotic fluid around him. His neck is elongating, so that his chin no longer rests on his chest. Head hair is developing and his finger- and toenails continue to grow.

Finer features

Baby's face is now better developed; all his features—eyes, ears, nose, and mouth—are recognizable, although his eyelids are still sealed shut. They will open at around 27 weeks.

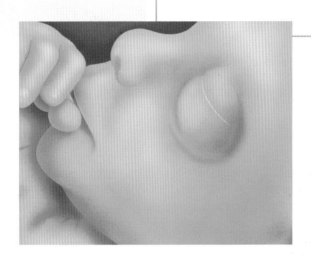

BABY'S LENGTH AND WEIGHT
His length, from crown to rump, will be around 3 to 3½ inches and he will weigh about .88 ounce.

Sign up for prenatal exercise class and set aside a day for light physical activity, such as swimming (see page 30).

DATES FOR YOUR DIARY

MONDAY	TUESDAY	WEDNESDAY	THURSDAY	FRIDAY	SATURDAY/SUNDAY

RELAXATION TECHNIQUES

Learning to relax is vital for you and for the well-being of your baby. It is also good preparation for dealing with the physical exertion of labor, when all your muscles will automatically tighten up in response to your uterine contractions and you will need to conserve energy and stay calm mentally.

Some women have difficulty sleeping when pregnant, despite feeling very tired. Even if you don't sleep, just lying down to rest with your eyes closed is beneficial. Daytime naps can help with overall fatigue, and getting regular exercise (see page 30) will help you sleep.

Muscular relaxation

Find somewhere quiet, comfortable, and warm to sit or lie down, then close your eyes. Start by tightening the muscles in your feet for a few seconds, then releasing them. Continue to work from your toes, feet, calves, thighs, buttocks, stomach, hands, and arms up to your face; tighten then release every muscle group in your body. Shut your eyes tightly and scrunch up your brow, then release. Open your jaw wide then release. Now repeat in reverse—work downward from your face. After this exercise your body should feel pleasantly heavy and limp. Practice this at least once a day for 10 or 20 minutes. Combine this with breathing exercises (see below) to intensify the relaxation.

Breathing techniques

It is a good idea to learn some deep breathing techniques while you are pregnant. Controlled breathing will help you relax and is invaluable during labor, both to deal with the pain and to keep you focused. Practice regular sessions of deep inhalations through your nose, followed by slow exhalations through your mouth (ten at a time). When you exhale, try to relax your muscles as well. Don't hold your breath—this makes you tense.

Meditation

Finding a sound or word to repeat, such as the word "relax," will allow you to block out external sensory input and clear your mind, resulting in mental and physical relaxation and revitalization. To benefit the most, practice meditation twice a day, for about 15 minutes a time, preferably at the same time.

If you can't find a particular word or phrase that works for you, try focusing on a happy memory or imaginary scene, such as lying on a beach or holding your newborn. Finding a quiet spot, turning off your cell phone, and lying or sitting with your eyes closed make the ideal setting for meditation.

Massage

In addition to the methods above, having a massage may also help you relax; ask a willing friend or partner to massage difficult-to-reach areas. Treating yourself to a professional back or full-body massage once in a while can be very rewarding.

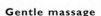

Gentle massage
Your partner can help you to relax by massaging aching feet or a painful neck or back.

Mom-to-be

By now your waistband is probably feeling tight, so it's time to think about looser-fitting maternity clothes (see page 38). Constipation may start to be a problem, due to increasing levels of progesterone, which cause the muscles of the intestine to slow, so eat plenty of fiber-rich fruit and vegetables and drink more water.

This week your baby's bones are growing rapidly, so make sure you keep up your calcium intake. See page 10 for information on getting vital nutrients from food.

If you're planning a vacation, the second trimester is the best time to go. Sex may also be back on the menu since many women find their libido heightened.

Baby

Starting from this week, extra-fine hair, called lanugo, starts to grow over her body, in intricate whorled patterns that follow the grain of her thin, translucent skin—patterns that will later give rise to fingerprints. Lanugo is thought to serve a protective function, acting as an anchor for the waxy skin covering that she will secrete in later months. It will be shed before birth and replaced by thicker, coarser hairs with which she will be born. Hair on her eyebrows and on her head also continues to grow.

The tiny bones of her middle ear are hardening, but she cannot yet hear properly. With facial muscles developing quickly now, she can make a range of expressions, such as frowning and grimacing.

Skeletal growth

Your baby is producing more bone and marrow, so she is becoming increasingly mobile and flexible. Her arms can now bend at the elbows and wrists and she can make fists.

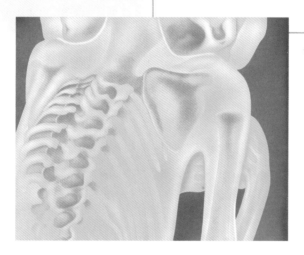

BABY'S LENGTH AND WEIGHT
Her length, from crown to rump, will be around 3⅔ to 4 inches and she will weigh about 1.75 ounces.

From about this week onward, an amniocentesis test may be scheduled (see page 36).

DATES FOR YOUR DIARY

MONDAY	TUESDAY	WEDNESDAY	THURSDAY	FRIDAY	SATURDAY/SUNDAY

FURTHER SCREENING TESTS

Though most doctors prefer to screen for risks of certain genetic diseases as early as possible, certain tests are only reliable later on in pregnancy.

Alpha-fetoprotein (AFP) and multiple marker

Between weeks 15 and 20, expectant mothers usually are offered a blood test called the multiple marker test. Sometimes called a triple screen or a quad screen, depending on the number of things measured, it also might be done in combination with blood tests and an ultrasound in the first trimester. For the multiple marker screening, a sample of blood is drawn from the mother to measure the levels of hCG (human chorionic gonadotropin), estriol, and alpha-fetoprotein (AFP). Sometimes the level of inhibin-A, which is made by the placenta, also is measured.

The levels of these substances can help doctors identify a fetus at risk for certain birth defects, including neural tube defects (like spina bifida) and some chromosomal abnormalities (like Down syndrome). In determining the results of the test, doctors take into account factors such as the mother's age, weight, and ethnicity, whether she has diabetes, if she is having twins or other multiples, and the age of the fetus. These variables can affect the levels of the substances being measured and can influence the interpretation of the test results, so the accuracy of this information is vital.

AMNIOCENTESIS

Samples of amniotic fluid can detect chromosomal abnormalities and the baby's sex, which is important if there is a familial propensity for a gender-based disorder. It is usually performed between weeks 15 and 20 and it carries a 0.5 percent risk of miscarriage. Under ultrasound monitoring, a thin, hollow needle is inserted through the abdomen into the amniotic sac. A small amount of fluid is drawn out to be analyzed. The results are available in about 7 to 10 days.

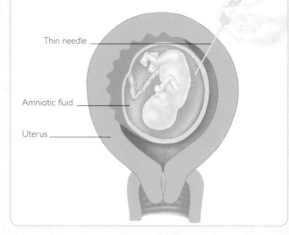

Thin needle

Amniotic fluid

Uterus

DOWN SYNDROME

Also known as Trisomy 21, this is a condition where a baby inherits an extra copy of chromosome 21 and, as a result, displays particular mental and physical characteristics. Anyone can give birth to a Down syndrome baby, but the risk does increase with a mother's age. The probability of giving birth to a baby with Down syndrome is one in 1,500 at 20 to 24 years old, one in 900 at 30 years old, one in 220 at 35 to 39 years old, and one in 100 at 40 years old.

Fluorescent in-situ hybridization

This test, also known as FISH, analyzes a small amount of amniotic fluid for major chromosomal abnormalities, with the results available within 24 to 48 hours. You can therefore rule out the majority of defects and find out the gender of your baby within 1 to 2 days. However, the amniotic fluid is still cultured, so final results will be ready in about a week.

Mom-to-be

Your uterus is expanding to make room both for your growing baby and placenta and the increasing amount of amniotic fluid—about 6¾ fluid ounces at this stage. Week 16 is an important week for testing: this is when AFP tests and other screenings are usually carried out (see page 36).

In preparation for breastfeeding, your milk glands start production now, which causes swelling and tenderness. Blood flow to the breasts increases, causing veins to become visible and the areolar glands (tiny bumps around the nipples) more pronounced.

Baby

Enough calcium has been deposited for the baby's bones to show up on an X-ray and his limbs are fully formed, with his legs growing longer than his arms. All his joints "work" and he can move everything—even bringing up his thumb to his mouth.

His head is more erect and his brain has taken more control of his nervous system and muscles, making each movement more deliberate, rapid, and complex. His immune system is starting to produce its own protective antibodies, taking over this role from his mother.

Little acrobat

Now your baby has the space and the ability to try out a wide range of movements. Kicks, somersaults, stretches, twists, turns, wriggles, and punches are all attempted, though probably undetected by you.

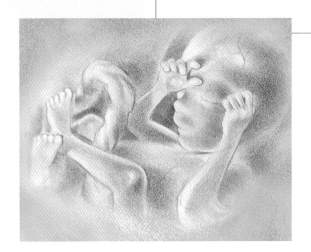

BABY'S LENGTH AND WEIGHT
His length, from crown to rump, will be around 4¼ to 4½ inches and he weighs about 2.8 ounces.

You may be scheduled for an AFP and multiple marker test this week.

DATES FOR YOUR DIARY

MONDAY	TUESDAY	WEDNESDAY	THURSDAY	FRIDAY	SATURDAY/SUNDAY

MATERNITY CLOTHES

As your bump starts to grow, you will need to find clothing to accommodate it, and with the huge variety in maternity clothing, there is no reason to lose your sense of style while pregnant.

Before rushing out to buy a whole new wardrobe, have a look through the clothes you own already. Any loose-fitting shirts, T-shirts, sweaters, or dresses may accommodate an expanding waistline. When your belly becomes more prominent, look for pants or skirts with drawstrings or elastic waistbands that sit above or below your bump. Maternity tops and dresses are the most accommodating for a growing belly and can be layered with a cardigan.

Maternity clothes can often be expensive, so it is worth asking recently pregnant friends and relatives of similar pre-pregnancy sizes if they have any spare maternity clothing.

Shopping for maternity clothes

Most maternity clothes are labeled according to your pre-pregnant size. If you are buying clothes from the nonmaternity section, it is best to try on items that are two sizes larger than what you usually wear; you can always add a belt, if necessary.

In all cases, choose clothes that are comfortable and easy to wear. Pregnant women tend to perspire more because of the increase in blood flow, so choose clothes made from natural fibers, such as cotton, wool, or linen, which allow your skin to breathe.

Maternity and nursing bras

A good-quality bra is essential early on in pregnancy. Your breasts start to enlarge very quickly and, if they don't have adequate support, the fibrous tissue will stretch, causing your breasts to sag, and possibly resulting in stretch marks (see page 46).

Your bra size may well change more than once during your pregnancy, so don't overbuy any one size. It's best to find a bra with at least three adjustment hooks, so that it grows with you. Ensure the straps are wide and the cups soft. Do not wear underwire bras because these can be uncomfortable for growing breasts. Above all, your bra should be as comfortable as possible, so enlisting the help of a store's trained bra-fitter is wise. If you have very large breasts, you may find it more comfortable to wear a bra 24 hours a day, possibly using a softer nursing sleep bra at night.

Footwear

Wear comfortable, low-heeled shoes that you can slip on rather than ones with laces or buckles. Later in your pregnancy, bending down will get more difficult, so loafers are best.

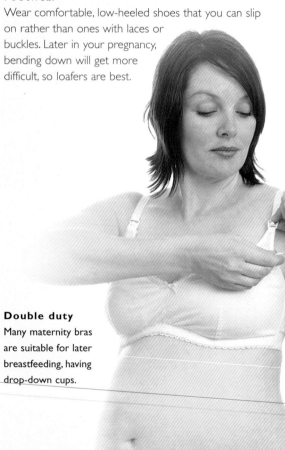

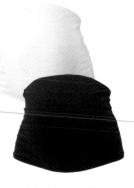

Belly bands
Made of thin, lightly elasticated fabric, these bands come in a variety of colors and styles. They sit comfortably on top of your bump and cover flesh exposed when your nonmaternity tops start to rise.

Double duty
Many maternity bras are suitable for later breastfeeding, having drop-down cups.

Mom-to-be

To meet the demands of your baby—and the placenta that feeds and cares for her—your heart has increased its output by roughly 40 percent. This greater volume of blood puts pressure on small blood vessels, such as the capillaries in your nose and gums, so be prepared for minor nosebleeds (and possibly a feeling of congestion) and bleeding gums. You may need to find a bigger bra by this stage and you may find your hands and feet swell a little due to water retention (edema).

Keep eating healthily because your baby requires as many nutrients as possible.

Baby

The major step this week is the deposition of brown fat, a special type of fat that will play a big role in heat generation after birth.

Her circulatory and urinary systems are working efficiently now and her heart pumps up to 25 quarts of blood a day. Her head is now more in proportion to her body; hair continues to grow on her head and face and eyelashes lengthen.

Matching the incredible growth rate of your baby is that of the placenta. This vital organ develops in tandem with the fetus, from the fingerlike projections of the villi in the first weeks, to a mass of tissue 1 inch in thickness and weighing more than 1 pound at full term. By week 17 it is large and well established, with a dense network of blood vessels, giving a huge surface area over which to exchange nutrients and waste products.

Delicate complexion
Your baby's skin is still very thin because there is no subcutaneous fat to flesh it out as yet. Underneath her eyelids her eyes have grown larger. Her fingers are very well developed and she can do a lot with them.

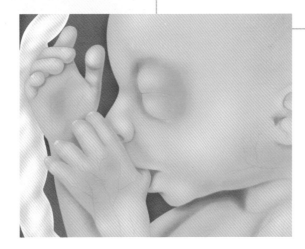

BABY'S LENGTH AND WEIGHT
Her length, from crown to rump, will be around 4 to 4¾ inches and she will weigh about 3.5 ounces.

 The results of your amniocentesis test may be back by now.

DATES FOR YOUR DIARY

MONDAY	TUESDAY	WEDNESDAY	THURSDAY	FRIDAY	SATURDAY/SUNDAY

SKIN, HAIR, NAILS, AND TEETH

Pregnancy hormones often result in a facial "glow"; skin and nails improve in condition and hair becomes shinier. However, for some women, the high levels of hormones coursing through them may result in more unwelcome body changes.

Skin

Most pregnant women are affected by darkened pigmentation on some area of their body. Body parts already pigmented, such as the areolas around your nipples and any freckles, may become more pronounced. A dark line, the linea nigra, may appear down the center of your abdomen. Although the pigmentation in these areas may stay dark for some time after your baby is born, the coloration will gradually fade.

Dilation of skin capillaries gives rise to spider naevi—raised red marks surrounded by spidery lines. They are caused by elevated estrogen levels and higher blood pressure, which dilate the tiny blood vessels in your skin and cause them to burst. Red palms (palmar erythema) is a related condition. Both of these will fade with time.

Some women find that irregular patches of brown skin appear on their forehead, cheeks, nose, and neck. Called chloasma or more commonly the "mask of pregnancy," it is caused by deeper skin pigmentation. Chloasma is exacerbated by sun exposure, so always use plenty of sunblock. It usually fades after birth.

Hair

If you're lucky, your hair will increase in thickness, growth, and shine. However, some women find that their hair becomes greasy or brittle and falls out in greater amounts. To combat dryness, use conditioner regularly; to prevent breakage, do not brush your hair too vigorously. If hair loss is noticeable, ask your hairdresser about a possible change in style. Your hair will improve again after pregnancy.

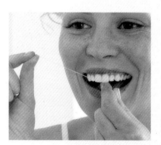

Teeth

During pregnancy, the gums soften and are more likely to bleed, making you more prone to infection. Ensure that your diet contains plenty of calcium and use an antibacterial mouthwash, if necessary. Go to the dentist regularly, but tell him or her you are pregnant so no X-rays are taken.

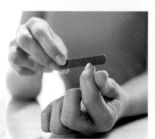

Nails

A common and welcome side effect of pregnancy is that fingernails usually grow stronger, faster, and thicker. But if you are unlucky and find your nails get brittle or thin, just keep your hands moisturized and nails cut short.

Mom-to-be

If you're pregnant for the first time, this week can be very exciting because it is around now that you may first feel your baby's movements. Many first-time mothers, however, may not feel any fetal movements until a few weeks later and especially if they are overweight.

Because of the increasing size of your abdomen, you may start to suffer from hemorrhoids around this week (see page 48). Eating foods high in fiber can help to prevent them and you can ask your healthcare provider or pharmacist about topical creams and ointments to ease discomfort.

Your growing bump may be starting to affect your balance, so take extra care and maintain good posture (see page 32).

Baby

He is more sensitive to the outside world now and signals his presence by means of kicks and prods. His hands can make fists and he should be able to hear because the part of his brain that receives and processes nerve signals from the ears is developing. He will become accustomed to the sound of blood rushing through the umbilical cord and of your heart beating, but will be startled by any loud noises.

Alveoli (air sacs) are developing in his fast-growing lungs, pads have formed on his fingers and toes, and rudimentary fingerprints are apparent. His eyes are in their final position, although still closed, and his face has fleshed out. His lower bowel is gathering undigested debris, called meconium, from swallowed amniotic fluid; this will form his first bowel movement.

If a boy, his prostate is forming.

Little sleepy head
Although he is rarely awake, your baby does have periods of activity when he is able to sense more of the outside world, as well as other parts of his body, even grabbing hold of his umbilical cord.

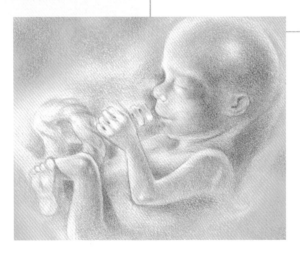

BABY'S LENGTH AND WEIGHT
His length, from crown to rump, will be around 5 to 5½ inches and he will weigh about 5.29 ounces.

At your next appointment with your healthcare provider, ask if you can listen to your baby's heartbeat.

DATES FOR YOUR DIARY

MONDAY	TUESDAY	WEDNESDAY	THURSDAY	FRIDAY	SATURDAY/SUNDAY

COMMUNICATING WITH YOUR BABY

You don't have to wait until your baby is born to establish a relationship with her—bonding and communication can begin while she is still in the uterus. At your very first ultrasound scan (see page 26), you may find yourself experiencing strong feelings of closeness to your growing baby, and starting from about week 18, this maternal-fetal bond grows stronger as your baby becomes familiar with your body rhythms, such as when you eat and sleep, and can be easily affected by your moods. This is why it is important to relax, stay calm, and be positive.

Your baby is also very sensitive to external stimuli, so if stroking your abdomen, do so gently. She will also benefit from hearing you and your partner talk to her, or if you sing or play music. Babies who have frequently heard their parents' voices in the womb are more easily soothed by them after birth.

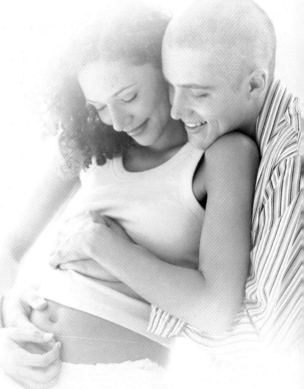

Fetal movements
Feeling your baby move for the first time is an affirmation of your pregnancy, and therefore a very exciting moment. Although fetal movements can rarely be felt before 14 weeks, most first-time mothers feel them between 18 and 22 weeks. However, because

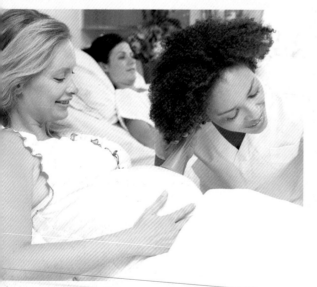

Hearing your baby's heartbeat
From as early as week 14 of pregnancy, a stethoscope or a sonic device can be used to hear your baby's heartbeat.

Fetal bonding
Both you and your partner will enjoy the sensations felt on the surface of your abdomen caused by your baby's movements. Stroking your stomach will reassure your baby.

some fetal movements feel like gentle stomach rumblings or butterflies, some first-time mothers might not even be able to identify them until around week 26. Your baby will have her own unique way of moving: some babies are extremely active, others make much more limited movements. As well as obvious kicks and prods, you may be able to feel your baby hiccupping.

As your baby grows, she will take up more of the available space until there is little left in which she can move. If she moves continuously in the same areas, such as under your ribs, this can cause you discomfort. If the pattern of movements changes suddenly, particularly if they decrease in frequency or intensity, consult your healthcare provider.

Mom-to-be

By now you may be feeling "quickening," the name for your baby's first discernible movements. Other changes include your pattern of weight gain; you may be gaining weight in certain areas, like the buttocks and hips, in addition to the abdomen. Your bigger uterus, together with your extra weight, is probably now affecting your posture, gait, and ability to sleep. Try using more pillows for support and to secure a more comfortable position at night.

Baby

Brain growth continues apace. Nerves connecting the muscles to the brain (motor neurons) have grown in place so that baby's movements are now consciously directed. Moreover, these movements are smoother and more coordinated because an insulating fatty nerve coating, known as myelin, has started to grow and promotes the smooth, rapid exchange of information. Your baby's skin has started to thicken, developing four layers.

Specialized sebaceous glands begin to secrete vernix caseosa, a waxy substance, also called vernix. This is a protective, waterproof barrier for fragile fetal skin, which is continuously immersed in amniotic fluid. Any imbibed amniotic fluid is now helped to pass into her circulation for filtering by gastric juices being produced in her gut.

Now, her ears stand out from the sides of her head, permanent tooth buds appear behind the ones for her deciduous (baby) teeth and her limbs are in proportion. Her nipples have appeared and genitalia are recognizable.

Uterine plaything

It is very common to see on an ultrasound scan a fetus grasping her umbilical cord. The thick and knotted texture of this resilient lifeline may provide baby with a variety of sensations that stimulate her sense of touch.

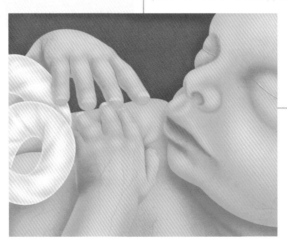

BABY'S LENGTH AND WEIGHT
Her length, from crown to rump, will be around 5 to 6 inches and she will weigh about 7 ounces.

You will probably have a detailed ultrasound scan this week or the next to check fetal anatomy.

DATES FOR YOUR DIARY

MONDAY	TUESDAY	WEDNESDAY	THURSDAY	FRIDAY	SATURDAY/SUNDAY

If you choose to, there is no reason why you should not continue working throughout your pregnancy. It is also a good way to keep busy and take your mind off the long wait. You may find, however, that you need to adjust your work routine for the sake of your own and your baby's well-being.

Safeguarding your health

Different jobs may have certain risks associated with them. For example, research has suggested that very hard physical activity may be associated with a slightly increased risk of compromised fetal growth. Other jobs may pose a risk by exposing a pregnant woman to hazardous substances. A hair stylist, for example, should spend minimal time working with dyes and hair spray and focus on other tasks such as shampooing or cutting.

If your work involves long hours spent on your feet, you may have to review the situation since backaches are a common pregnancy complaint. Night-shift work may also have to be reviewed because sleep is increasingly important as pregnancy develops.

Work station setup

If you sit at a desk all day, you may be at a greater risk of developing a blood clot, so discuss your specific work situation with your healthcare provider. If you work in front if a computer screen all day, take frequent breaks to get up and move around. Make sure your work station is set up properly: sit in a height-adjustable chair with a back rest, wrist support, and footstool. When sitting, keep your feet raised as often as possible.

Maternity Leave

This is the time a mother takes off from work for the birth of a child. It is also known as parental or family leave because sometimes fathers take leave as well. Parents are protected by the Family and Medical Leave Act (FMLA) of 1993, which mandated 12 weeks job-protected medical leave to mothers to attend to a newborn child. As well as being unpaid time off, there are a number of limiting stipulations, and the act does not cover those who work for smaller companies. To be eligible under the FMLA, you must work in a firm of 50 or more employees, be employed by the same business for 12 months, and have accumulated at least 1,250 working hours over those 12 months. Certain states have supplemented the federal regulations and have extended maternity leave benefits. However, in most cases, you'll use a combination of short-term disability (STD), sick leave, vacation, personal days, and unpaid family leave during your time away from work. Which benefits are available to you will depend very much on which state you live in. For example, not all states allow women to take short-term disability leave to cover pregnancy, birth, and postpartum recovery.

In 2002, California led the way in enacting paid family leave, and other states such as Washington and New Jersey followed suit. Some enlightened companies now offer parents paid time off—as many as six weeks in some cases—but paid leave is highly unusual in the US. Check the regulations in your state and at your place of work because your employer may have policies that dictate the order in which you can take different kinds of leave. Whatever the situation, you'll want to start investigating your options as early as you can during your pregnancy and make sure you have all your paperwork in order before the baby arrives.

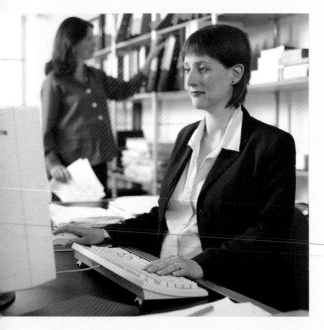

Supportive work station
As the weeks go by and your bump grows, you will need to adjust your work station in order to sit comfortably in front of your computer.

Mom-to-be

It is now 18 weeks since conception and you will look noticeably pregnant. Your waistline has expanded considerably so that it is no longer visible and your uterus is pushing your abdomen outward. At this time, the top of your uterus (fundus) should be just below your navel.

If you have a scan this week, you may well be able to hear the sound of your baby's heartbeat through a stethoscope or Doppler ultrasound—a truly breathtaking experience.

Baby

Now midway into his growth, this time is crucial for baby's sensory development.

More vernix is being produced, anchored in place by the downy lanugo hairs, and is particularly thick around the eyebrows. His skin is thickening and is now made up of four layers, one of which contains epidermal ridges which are responsible for the surface patterns on fingertips, palms of the hands, and soles of the feet. Toenails are beginning to grow and scalp hair continues to appear.

If a girl, she now has around six million eggs in her ovaries (though only one million will still be there at birth).

Vital brain development

More of the nerve cells required for the five senses—sight, taste, smell, hearing, and touch—have developed. Also increasing are the complex synapses (neurological connections) required for memory and thinking.

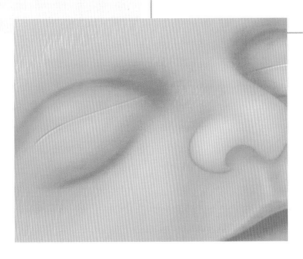

BABY'S LENGTH AND WEIGHT
His length, from crown to rump, will be around 5½ to 6¼ inches and he will weigh about 9 ounces.

You may be having your anomaly scan or ultrasound level two scan this week (see page 36).

DATES FOR YOUR DIARY

MONDAY	TUESDAY	WEDNESDAY	THURSDAY	FRIDAY	SATURDAY/SUNDAY

COMMON COMPLAINTS

The hormonal and physical changes your body undergoes during pregnancy can lead to a variety of physical complaints, the majority of which may be uncomfortable, but are generally not serious. The chart on the right has solutions to some of the most common problems.

Your changing hormone levels can also result in mood swings, including feelings of irritability and anxiety. Controlled breathing and meditation are two effective ways of relaxing and calming the mind (see page 34). In addition, mood swings may be a result of, or accompanied by, insomnia.

Stretch marks

Though not an inevitable result of pregnancy, many women find they develop stretch marks on their stomachs, hips, and breasts. These red or brown streaks are the result of a sudden gain in weight. When you gain a lot of weight in a short space of time, your skin doesn't have the chance to adapt and it stretches to accommodate your new shape. While these marks will gradually fade to a silvery sheen, there are things you can do to help prevent them appearing in the first place. The first is to avoid gaining too much weight; if you eat sensibly, this shouldn't be a problem. Keep your skin supple by massaging cocoa butter or almond oil extract into your breasts, hips, and stomach. Make sure your breasts are adequately supported; wear a well-fitting bra and, if your breasts are large, wear a sleep bra at night.

Swollen hands, feet, and ankles

Normal body fluids increase in pregnancy and about 75 percent of pregnant women will develop edema (swelling) at some time. It is most notable at the end of the day, in warmer weather, or after prolonged standing and sitting. To help prevent water retention, wear loose-fitting clothing and loafers and remove any tight bracelets or rings. Don't stand or sit for too long in one position. Sudden swelling may signal preeclampsia (see page 58); if this happens, seek medical help urgently.

PROBLEM	WHAT TO DO
Backache	Ask your partner or a friend to massage your lower back. Wear low-heeled shoes throughout your pregnancy and always pay attention to your posture, especially when lifting objects from the floor (see page 32).
Constipation	Drink at least eight 8-ounce glasses of fluid a day (avoid fruit juice, which is high in sugar). Eat plenty of high-fiber foods, fresh vegetables and fruit, and wholegrain cereals. Frequent exercise (see page 30) will stimulate the digestive tract.
Dizziness	Sit on a chair and bend over so your head is between your knees. When lying down, keep your feet raised higher than your head.
Heartburn	Avoid overfilling your stomach by eating little and often, instead of three large meals. Talk to your healthcare provider about safe antacid remedies.
Leg Cramps	To help ease the pain, walk around with bare feet and try stretching and extending your legs and feet. Giving your legs a massage can also help.
Gas and Bloating	Avoid eating large meals that may leave you feeling bloated and uncomfortable. Don't rush your meals; this can cause you to swallow air, which can cause painful pockets of gas.
Varicose Veins	Rest and elevate your legs and feet as much as possible and massage gently around the area—not directly on the veins. Wear compression stockings.
Breathlessness	Try not to panic if you can't catch your breath—this can make matters worse. Stand tall and allow your chest plenty of room to expand. Try to relax as much as possible and avoid situations you know to be stressful. If you begin to wheeze, experience chest pain, or if your fingers and lips turn blue, seek medical advice urgently.

Mom-to-be

Your weight begins to increase more rapidly over the next ten weeks as your baby lays down her fat layers. This weight gain will be about half your total gain. You may also notice an increase in your appetite, prompted by the extra calories you need to support your increased basal metabolism. Continue to eat well but avoid bingeing on one or two foods alone, and unhealthy and fatty snacks with little nutritional value.

Don't be surprised if you experience a craving for something uncommon. This is known as pica, and soot and soil are among some of the more unusual things women have been known to have a strong desire for.

Varicose veins (see page 46) are a potential problem now, so minimize the risk by wearing compression stockings, exercising daily, and elevating your legs as much as possible.

Baby

Weight gain continues this week, which is vital for keeping her warm after birth. Her digestive system is now advanced enough to absorb water and sugars from the amniotic fluid that she swallows, filtering some of it through the kidneys and passing what little solid matter there is as far as the large bowel. What her kidneys can't remove is redirected via the placenta to your bloodstream and kidneys. Taste buds are starting to form on her tongue and her sense of touch is improved due to brain and nerve-ending development. On a scan she may be seen stroking her face, sucking her thumb, or playing with her umbilical cord.

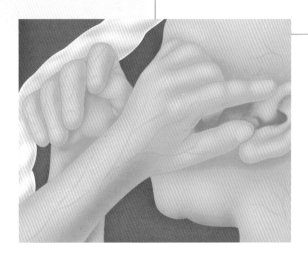

Sound equipment

Hearing is a feature from early in pregnancy; the uterus is not a quiet place. Your baby hears your voice—including sneezes and coughs, your heartbeat, your organs, and circulation "working," and any hiccups you may make. Soon, your baby will listen all the time.

BABY'S LENGTH AND WEIGHT
Her length, from crown to rump, will be around 7 inches and she will weigh about 10.5 ounces.

 This could be a good time to buy a baby name book.

DATES FOR YOUR DIARY

MONDAY	TUESDAY	WEDNESDAY	THURSDAY	FRIDAY	SATURDAY/SUNDAY

MORE COMMON COMPLAINTS

Difficulty sleeping

Anxieties about the baby's well-being as well as physical discomforts can result in sleepless nights. To help ensure a good night's sleep, have a soothing aromatic bath using a little lavender oil before going to bed. Make sure your bedroom is neither too warm nor too cool and always wear lightweight, unrestrictive nightwear, preferably in natural fibers. Spend time outdoors so you get plenty of fresh air. Don't eat a heavy meal before bed but try a warm drink of camomile tea or milk, which are known for their soporific effects.

Hemorrhoids

Many pregnant women suffer from hemorrhoids, usually from around week 18 of pregnancy. Hemorrhoids are swollen (varicose) veins, which appear inside the rectum and may protrude through the anus. They are caused by your growing uterus bearing down on your rectum. The increased pressure impedes the flow of blood in the veins. The veins then dilate to accommodate the trapped blood. The area around your anus may become sore and itchy and you may also notice bleeding when passing stools. To relieve itching, apply an ice pack or some soothing ointment or cream recommended by your healthcare provider. Hemorrhoids usually shrink and disappear after delivery.

Frequency of urination

Your growing baby will put pressure on your bladder, which can make you need to urinate more frequently or even leak urine—particularly when you laugh or sneeze. Pelvic floor exercises will help prevent leakage and

PELVIC FLOOR (KEGEL) EXERCISES

A group of muscles support the openings to the urethra, vagina, and rectum. Specially designed exercises will help tone these muscles, enabling them to support your growing baby's weight and helping to push him out during delivery. Keeping these muscles in shape will also help you recover more quickly after the birth. Kegel (named after the doctor who developed them) exercises can be done anywhere, anytime, and without any special equipment.

To perform Kegel exercises, simply tighten your pelvic floor muscles, hold for a count of five (increasing to 10, 15, etc.) then slowly release. It can help to imagine your muscles as an elevator going up. To make the "elevator" descend, gradually relax the muscles. Repeat as often as possible.

wearing light sanitary or incontinence pads will catch any leaks. Although you may be inclined to, don't cut back on your fluid intake because this can cause constipation (see page 46). Urine loss can be a sign of a urinary tract infection and a continuous loss of fluid may be a sign of ruptured membranes; in both cases, seek medical advice.

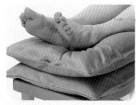

Leg and calf cramps

A firm massage will relieve painful cramps in your calf or thigh. When standing, pull up your foot from the toes and push down into the heel. Briskly rub the calf. If you tend to suffer from frequent cramps, you may be lacking in calcium or salt.

Aching legs

Sit in a comfortable chair and elevate your feet as often as possible. Try wearing compression stockings or massaging your legs.

Mom-to-be

Your increased blood volume has the effect of diluting your blood to give what is known as the "physiological anemia of pregnancy." Physiological anemia is common, but your healthcare provider will determine if you are getting enough iron. You can increase your iron intake by eating red meat, bran, sesame seeds, and lentils, accompanied by a small glass of orange juice to aid iron absorption.

Your growing uterus can put pressure on your lungs, stomach, and bladder, which can result in breathlessness upon exertion, indigestion, and the need to urinate more frequently. Stretch marks may appear on your abdomen, breasts, and hips (see page 46).

Now comfortably into your pregnancy, you can think about taking a break and going away for the weekend before your bump becomes too big.

Baby

His brain continues to grow very quickly, especially in the area where brain cells are produced, and his internal organs are becoming more specialized in their individual tasks.

Even though he is still red and wrinkled and covered in lanugo, his skin is less transparent and he has developed sweat glands. His fingernails are now fully formed and continue to grow.

Patterns of sleep and wakefulness can now be recorded and your baby is more aware. He can be woken if you tap on your abdomen, by loud noise, or by sudden movement. When sucking his thumb, he can either bring his thumb to his mouth or bend his head to his hand. This learning process is repeated after birth, when he will integrate the tactile knowledge he has gained in the uterus with information from his eyes (and from putting things in his mouth).

Gender characteristics

If a boy, your baby's testes are descending from his pelvis to his scrotum and primitive sperm are forming. If a girl, her vagina is beginning to hollow.

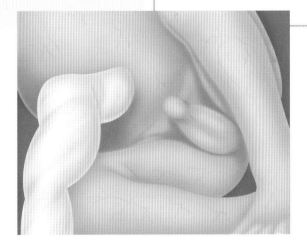

BABY'S LENGTH AND WEIGHT
His length, from crown to rump, will be around 7½ inches and he will weigh about 12 ounces.

Think about booking a pregnancy massage or pedicure to give yourself a lift!

DATES FOR YOUR DIARY

MONDAY	TUESDAY	WEDNESDAY	THURSDAY	FRIDAY	SATURDAY/SUNDAY

MAINTAINING INTIMACY

Sex during pregnancy—penetrative or otherwise—can increase the sense of love, intimacy, and sharing between partners. Many women find they have an increased sexual desire during their pregnancy, particularly during the second trimester. This is mainly due to the huge increase in sex hormones (a mixture of estrogen and progesterone) that start circulating around the body from the moment of conception. As well as heightened sensual feelings, these hormones are also responsible for your hair and skin changes (see page 40). A pregnant woman's blood flow also increases, particularly around the pelvic region, and this makes her genitals more sensitive and easier to arouse. Sex during pregnancy can sometimes be far more exciting than normal and a woman may even achieve orgasm for the first time.

Most men find a partner's changing body extremely attractive. However, there are some men who find the thought of intercourse unsettling because they worry about harming their partner or baby.

Unless otherwise advised by your healthcare provider, there is no physiological reason why you should abstain from sex during pregnancy. Your baby is encased in amniotic fluid, which protects her from any bumps or bruising, and the cervical mucus, which plugs the entrance to the uterus, prevents any bacterial infections from entering. However, there are things you can do to make the experience more comfortable.

Sex in the "missionary" position should be avoided after four months; a side-lying or woman-on-top position will allow you to better control the depth of penetration. A lubricant can help prevent soreness and abrasions, and thrusting should be kept to a minimum.

There are also alternatives to full penetrative sex that may be enjoyed by both partners—extended foreplay, sensual massage, mutual masturbation, and oral sex, for example. Sharing a bath, kissing, and cuddling are other ways of showing affection.

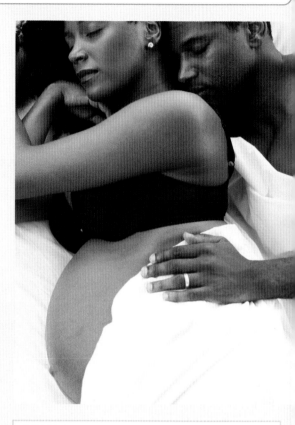

STAY SAFE

Although generally there is no risk to your unborn baby when you make love, you may want to avoid penetrative sex until you are beyond the first 12 weeks if you have a history of miscarriages. You may also want to avoid it in the last trimester if you previously had a premature delivery or are experiencing signs of early labor. You should also avoid sex in late pregnancy if your membranes have broken or if you have any bleeding.

Mom-to-be

Your growing abdomen may be impacting on your digestive system, causing heartburn and indigestion. Eating smaller, more frequent meals can help, as can walking after eating. This may be the time when you start to suffer from anemia, so it's important to eat plenty of iron-rich foods.

Braxton Hicks contractions may start about now. These irregular and painless contractions are part of your uterus' training for labor. As your pregnancy advances, they will get stronger, but do not mistake them for true labor. You can feel them if you put your hand on your abdomen, but otherwise they may pass unnoticed.

Talk to your baby. She can hear well now and will respond to various sounds.

Baby

Her face and body look more like a full-term baby now, but her bones and organs are still visible beneath the skin.

Although she is laying down fat at a high rate, she looks wrinkled because skin is being produced faster than the subcutaneous fat that fills it out, so the skin hangs loosely.

Her lips are much more pronounced and her deciduous (milk) teeth buds sit below her gum line. Her eyes—still fused shut—are formed, but the irises lack pigment.

Her pancreas is developing steadily; later it will supply insulin, an important hormone for maintaining fat in her tissues.

Her hearing is more acute since the ear bones have hardened; she can hear deeper male voices more easily than higher-pitched female ones.

Color change

Your baby's skin now appears red because pigment is starting to be laid down, making the skin color less translucent.

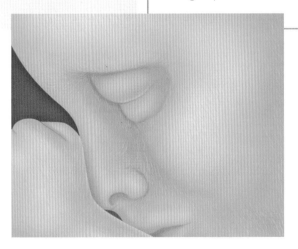

BABY'S LENGTH AND WEIGHT
Her length, from crown to rump, will be around 8 inches and she will weigh about 16 ounces.

If you are working, talk to your supervisor and the Human Resources department to finalize your maternity leave plans.

DATES FOR YOUR DIARY

MONDAY	TUESDAY	WEDNESDAY	THURSDAY	FRIDAY	SATURDAY/SUNDAY

SELECTING BABY EQUIPMENT

Whether you buy new or used equipment, make sure that all items meet or exceed US safety standards. Children's products are subject to a set of federal safety rules, called Children's Product Safety Rules.

Feeding equipment

For both breast- and bottlefeeding you will need small bottles, rings, nipples and caps, a bottle brush, and a sterilizer. For breastfeeding, you will also need a battery-operated breast pump to express milk, and some breast pads.

Diapers

With cloth diapers, you will need plastic pants, diaper liners (inserts), and safety pins (unless the diapers are self-fastening using snaps). You will also need two buckets—one for soiled diapers and one for urine-soaked ones. For disposables, you need disposable diaper bags and a garbage can with a lid.

Buggy, stroller, or sling

Buggies are the best, but most expensive, option for newborns. Sturdy, covered, and with added suspension for a smooth ride and to make them easy to push, buggies are padded for comfort. The baby lies in the buggy facing the pusher. A stroller, which is an open, folding device, is only suitable for babies from three months of age. The baby sits in the stroller facing the direction of travel. Rugged three-wheeled "jogging strollers" are also very popular.

A baby sling or soft fabric carrier will enable you to hold the baby close to your chest. There are many different styles, but the important thing is that the sling does not interfere with baby's breathing, so the baby's face, nose, and mouth must be visible at all times. The item should carry a US safety standards logo.

Car seat

This must be suitable for a newborn and should carry a safety standards logo and ideally have a 5-point safety harness. It must be installed rearward-facing back seat, and not in a seat fitted with an airbag. Child passenger restraint laws vary by state to so check local regulations.

Bed and bedding

For the first few weeks your baby can sleep in a bassinet or Moses basket. Later, he will need a separate crib with bars spaced no more than 2 inches apart so he cannot put his head through them. The crib should have a drop-down side with a safety catch. If buying a used crib, ensure that the woodwork is smooth with no splinters, and the paint or varnish is nontoxic. Buy a snug-fitting waterproof mattress. You will need at least three fitted sheets. To avoid Sudden Infant Death Syndrome (SIDS), product safety experts advise against using pillows, overly soft mattresses, sleep positioners, bumper pads, stuffed animals, or fluffy bedding in the crib and recommend instead dressing the child warmly and keeping the crib bare.

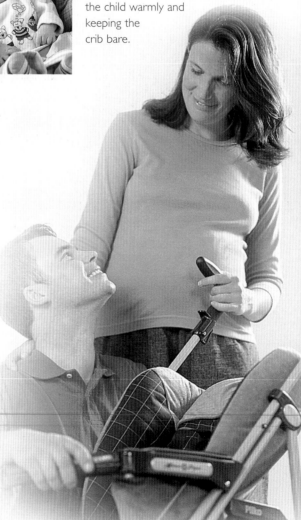

Mom-to-be

Your weight gain may be taking its toll and backache, bladder problems, sore feet, and general fatigue may all affect you from now on. So, it's a good idea to start organizing things to make your life as easy as possible. For instance, make sure that you continue to wear comfortable shoes and take every opportunity to put your feet up, raising them above the level of your heart if possible. Also, ask your partner, friends, and relatives to help with running errands.

You may have an prenatal appointment this week to check on your own and your baby's health.

Baby

This is a landmark week for your baby's growth because, if born now, he might survive. But he is still very thin with immature lungs and would face a wide range of difficulties. He would need to be kept in an incubator under expert care.

His head is still large in relation to the rest of his body, but his body continues to grow, filling the uterus and making his movements more restricted. He is building up fat but still has red, wrinkled skin, which is thicker on the soles and palms.

Increasingly conscious of the outside world because his hearing is well established, he can hear music, as well as your voice, your heartbeat, and stomach rumblings.

Importantly, he has begun producing surfactant, a substance vital in helping his lungs expand at birth by keeping the air sacs from sticking together.

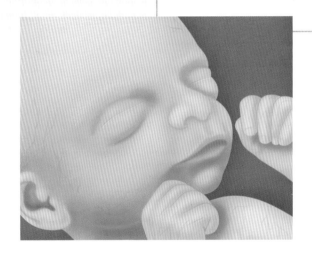

That's my baby!
Your baby's facial features are now more or less complete; his eyelashes and eyebrows are quite well developed and hair continues to grow on his scalp.

BABY'S LENGTH AND WEIGHT
His length, from crown to rump, will be around 8¼ inches and he will weigh about 19 ounces.

You should be booking, or at least investigating, childbirth education classes now.

DATES FOR YOUR DIARY

MONDAY	TUESDAY	WEDNESDAY	THURSDAY	FRIDAY	SATURDAY/SUNDAY

CHOOSING A LAYETTE SET

Selecting items for your baby's wardrobe can be great fun, though you should always remember that until your baby is born and her weight and measurements are known, it is best to buy only the immediate essentials. You can always buy more suitable clothing once she arrives. Bear in mind, too, that you may well receive clothing as gifts. In any event, avoid newborn sizes because all babies quickly outgrow these and the same is true when considering more expensive outfits; your baby may only wear them once!

The right choice

Clothes can quickly become dirty or stained, particularly in the diaper area and neckline, so they will need to be changed and washed frequently. Buy colorfast, machine-washable clothes that are also suitable for tumble-drying. Avoid synthetic fabrics, which can be scratchy against your baby's newborn skin; choose natural fabrics such as cotton and wool instead. Clothing made from organic bamboo fibers is also available. Check all garments for raised seams and scratchy labels (you may be able to remove these). Don't buy anything that needs hand washing or ironing.

If you don't know the sex of your baby or you don't want to adhere to the stereotype of dressing girls in pink and boys in blue, buy items in gender-neutral colors such as yellow, green, or white and patterns, such as stripes, plaid, teddy bears, or toy blocks.

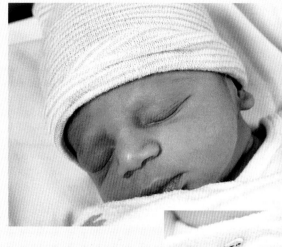

Until the birth, keep all clothes in the packaging and hang on to the receipts so you can exchange them if your baby is born prematurely or is born too large to wear them.

Once baby is here, make sure you wash her clothes before putting them on her the first time. They don't, however, need to be washed separately from your clothes and no special laundry detergent is required either.

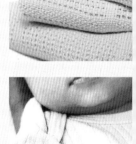

WHAT TO BUY

- 50 small-size disposable diapers (to start with) or 24 cloth diapers
- 4 bibs
- 5 short-sleeve lap shoulder undershirts
- 4 babygrows (sleepsuits or onesies)
- 3 infant gowns or sleepsacks
- 2 hooded baby towels
- 1 facecloth
- 2 cardigans
- 2 shawls
- 1 summer or winter hat
- 2 pairs socks or booties

Mom-to-be

Your uterus has grown to the size of a soccer ball, pushing your diaphragm and lower ribs up, and displacing your stomach. Pressure on your abdomen may cause your belly button to stick out, giving you an "outie" if previously you had an "innie." Together with the effects of progesterone, which slows down the emptying of food from the stomach, the pressure on your stomach means that you are much more likely to back up acid into the esophagus (lower throat) and get heartburn, particularly after heavy meals.

Baby

She is now well proportioned, though still thin-skinned and skinny. Blood vessels continue to develop in her lungs and her other vital organs are now well developed.

High inside the gums, her permanent teeth are developing in buds and her nostrils are beginning to open. The nerves around her mouth and lips are more sensitive in preparation for breastfeeding and she practices by sucking on body parts.

Sex differentiation is complete: if your baby is a boy, his testes have descended into the scrotum; if a girl, the vagina has finished hollowing out.

Growth time

Your baby has settled into a daily pattern of sleep and activity. It is while sleeping that she develops, grows, and prepares for birth. While sleeping, her brain is working, producing rapid eye movements that can be recorded.

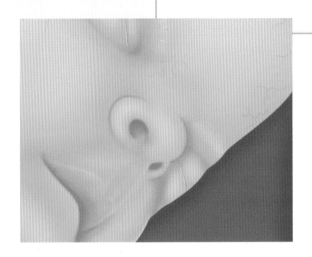

BABY'S LENGTH AND WEIGHT
Her length, from crown to rump, will be almost 9 inches and she will weigh about 1½ pounds.

See if you can make an appointment to tour the hospital or birth center so you can view the facilities.

DATES FOR YOUR DIARY

MONDAY	TUESDAY	WEDNESDAY	THURSDAY	FRIDAY	SATURDAY/SUNDAY

PREPARING YOUR BABY'S ROOM

For the first few weeks, your baby can sleep in a Moses basket or bassinet in your bedroom. This makes his frequent night feeds more convenient for you; it has also been suggested as a preventive measure for Sudden Infant Death Syndrome (SIDS). However, sooner rather than later your baby should have his own room in which he sleeps and where all his clothes and associated equipment are kept. Don't leave all the decorating to the last few weeks when you will tire easily.

Interior design

Most people will prepare a baby's room with the intention that he will live there for at least a few years. For this reason, it is important to decorate the nursery in a style that will be suitable when your baby is of toddler and preschool age. Research has indicated that babies prefer bold, primary colors and distinct patterns because they can focus on these much better than soft, pastel patterns. Buy an interestingly shaped or musical mobile to hang over your baby's crib, and large pictures of animals or friendly cartoon characters to put up on the walls.

Furniture

You will need a waist-high changing table with drawers to store diapers, wipes, and other cleaning products, as well as other storage units for baby's clothes and toys. Lamps, or a dimmer switch on the main light, are a good idea for night feeds, as is a comfortable rocking chair in which you can feed your baby. Buy a baby monitor, and make sure that your baby's room is adequately heated (around 68°F), well ventilated, and quiet.

Safety

The paint, fabrics, and floor coverings you use should be as environmentally friendly as possible. Avoid using any strong-smelling paints, wash curtains before hanging them, and have someone else remove any old carpet. Careful placement of furniture will make baby care safer and less tiring. Things should be within easy reach for parents, but out of harm's way for the baby. Place the crib and changing table against a wall and away from a window; ensure there are no dangling cords from blinds or curtains within reach of the baby.

To forestall problems when your baby starts to crawl, place childproof covers over electrical outlets, and cover any radiators with a protective guard.

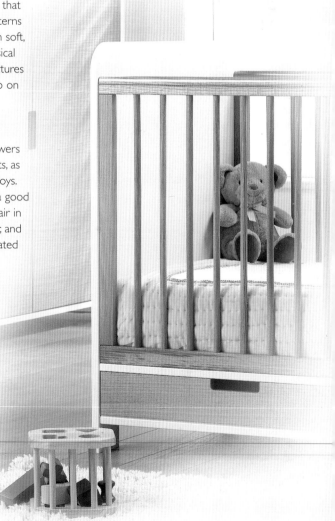

Mom-to-be

As you near the end of the second trimester, a number of new discomforts may appear. These include back pain, leg cramps, headaches, and pressure on and around your pelvis (see pages 56 and 58 for suggestions on easing these). In addition, your baby's movements may also occasionally cause pain beneath your ribs, which can be relieved if you lie on your side.

Dad may be able to hear your baby's heartbeat if he puts his head on your stomach. A scan at week 26 is a truly bonding experience because you can see your baby's profile, anatomy, facial expressions, and watch his movements.

Baby

Although the space in the uterus is becoming ever more restricted, he continues to grow. His spine is strong enough to support his body and he responds to touch and sound—his pulse quickens when he hears noise and he can move in rhythm to music. He continues to practice breathing movements and his lungs are maturing. His eyebrows are complete and while he still looks lean, fat is being deposited continuously. By the time he is born, his weight will have increased radically and he will emerge rounded and plump.

If a boy, the cells in your baby's testes have increased, which is important for testosterone production.

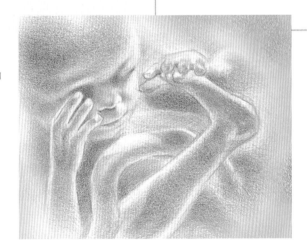

Touching toes
Your baby can probably hold his feet in his fist now. If he manages to get his feet into his mouth, he will suck on the toes.

BABY'S LENGTH AND WEIGHT
His length, from crown to rump, will be around 9 inches and he will weigh about nearly 2 pounds.

Discuss with your ideas and the options available for your birth plan (see page 93) with your healthcare provider.

DATES FOR YOUR DIARY

MONDAY	TUESDAY	WEDNESDAY	THURSDAY	FRIDAY	SATURDAY/SUNDAY

MEDICAL EMERGENCIES

Most pregnancies proceed without major complications, but things can go wrong, so it's important to be aware of the danger signs. Miscarriage, generally as a result of fetal chromosomal abnormalities, is a feature of early pregnancy, as is an ectopic pregnancy. The conditions below, while not common, generally affect pregnancy in the second and third trimesters.

Preeclampsia and eclampsia

Characterized by raised blood pressure, protein in the urine, and increased swelling of the legs and feet, preeclampsia affects 6 to 8 percent of pregnancies, and 85 percent of these are first-time pregnancies. As well as excessive weight gain, other warning signs are persistent headaches, flashing lights, blurred vision or spots in front of the eyes, or upper abdominal pain on the right side of the body. If you notice any of these symptoms, you should seek medical help urgently. Treatment is directed at lowering the blood pressure. In rare cases, preeclampsia can develop into eclampsia and urgent delivery of the baby is generally required.

Incompetent cervix

During pregnancy the entrance to the uterus, the cervix, is kept closed by a plug of mucus. Sometimes, however, the cervix starts to dilate before the pregnancy is complete due to the pressure of a growing uterus and baby. Known as an incompetent cervix, it can result in the amniotic sac sagging into the vaginal canal and breaking, which can bring on a miscarriage. Incompetent cervix is believed to be responsible for 20 to 25 percent of all second trimester miscarriages.

Securing the cervix
If your cervix opens early, your doctor will put a stitch (suture) in it for the duration of your pregnancy.

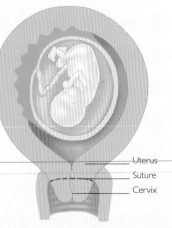

Uterus
Suture
Cervix

WARNING SIGNS

If you experience any of the following, seek medical help urgently:
- Unusual persistent abdominal or chest pain
- Excessive vomiting or diarrhea
- Headaches, flashing lights in front of the eyes, double vision
- Itching all over
- Leaking of blood or fluid from the vagina
- Swollen or painful leg
- Chills and fever
- Painful or burning urination
- Infrequent urination and thirst
- Seizures
- Fall
- Slowing or absence of fetal movements

If it is diagnosed in time, your doctor will put a stitch in your cervix to keep it closed and then remove it about a week before you are due. Women at higher risk of cervical incompetence include those carrying more than one baby, or those who have had a cone biopsy, cervical surgery, or laser therapy. In these cases, a doctor may recommend a vaginal ultrasound to check all is well.

Placenta previa

In about one in 200 pregnancies, the placenta lies at the bottom of the uterus instead of at the top. It moves out of the way 95 percent of the time as the uterus grows, but if it remains in an abnormal position, it can cause complications during delivery. If the placenta blocks the entrance to the uterus completely, a cesarean section (also called a C-section) will be necessary.

The main symptom of placenta previa is bright red bleeding, especially after week 28. If this occurs, seek medical advice urgently. An ultrasound scan will be needed to confirm the condition.

Mom-to-be

In late pregnancy the cholesterol levels in your blood rise, but this should not be a cause for concern. Cholesterol is a vital building block for various pregnancy hormones, which are manufactured by the placenta. These include progesterone, which is important for breast development and relaxation of the uterine and other smooth muscles.

Keep talking and singing to your baby because she knows your voice and will feel comforted by such communication.

Baby

With eye formation complete, her protective eyelashes are also fully grown. She is becoming plumper due to increased fat building under the skin and, if born now, would look almost the same as at full term, albeit a lot thinner and smaller. The taste buds on her tongue and inside her cheeks are fully functioning and she will enjoy sucking on anything that comes within range of her mouth.

Her lungs continue to grow and she would have a 90 percent chance of surviving if born now. However, she is far from fully developed and would have to be kept in an incubator, artificially respirated. Also, she would have inadequate liver function, an underdeveloped brain and a weak immune system, leaving her susceptible to the sort of infections that a full-term baby would shrug off with ease.

Eye spy...

The long development of the baby's eyes is now complete and her eyelids can open some of the time.

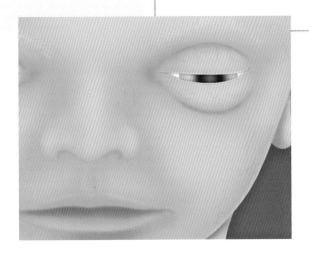

BABY'S LENGTH AND WEIGHT
Her length, from crown to rump, will be around 9½ inches and she will weigh about 2¼ pounds.

Shop for baby equipment and supplies before you get too big.

DATES FOR YOUR DIARY

MONDAY	TUESDAY	WEDNESDAY	THURSDAY	FRIDAY	SATURDAY/SUNDAY

PREPARING FOR A HOME BIRTH

Controversial decision

In the US, home birth remains contentious. The American College of Obstetricians and Gynecologists (ACOG) and the American Medical Association (AMA) oppose home birth and contend that the hospital is the safest place to give birth—capabilities of the hospital setting and the expertise of staff are immediately available if a complication arises suddenly. However, both the American College of Nurse-Midwives and the Governing Council of the American Public Health Association support the choice of women who are good candidates to give birth at home, as long as reliable backup and transfer arrangements are in place.

Legal issues

Look for a certified nurse-midwife, a certified direct-entry midwife, or a physician with plenty of experience of delivering babies at home. Ask about her education, her credentials, and whether she's licensed to practice in your state. The vast majority of direct-entry midwives are

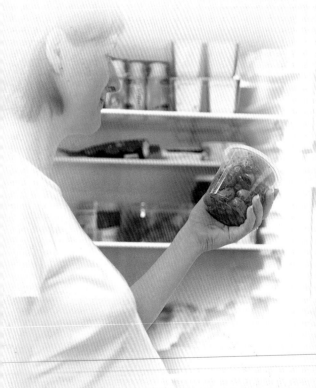

MIDWIFE'S REQUIREMENTS

- Easy access to the birth room and plenty of space both sides of the bed; parking for herself, and for the emergency services, if they should be needed.
- An area in which the midwife can place all of her equipment.
- Plenty of towels, facecloths, washbowls, and some soft towels or a shawl in which to wrap your newborn baby.

Certified Professional Midwives, specializing in birth outside of a hospital, particularly in private homes and at freestanding birth centers, and are the only birth attendants whose education and clinical training focuses specifically on out-of-hospital birth settings. Be aware, though, that in 23 states there are no licensing laws for direct-entry midwives (legislation is pending in 13 states at time of writing) and she can be arrested for practicing unlicensed. In all 50 states, it is legal, however, to hire a Certified Nurse-Midwife, though most work in hospitals.

Protecting your home

Because there will be a lot of amniotic fluid and some bloody discharge during the birth, you will need protective coverings for the bed or sofa and the surrounding floor. Alternatively, you can use old sheets, tablecloths, and newspapers. You should also stock up on large plastic garbage bags to make cleaning up easier.

Comfort

In the bedroom, gather as many pillows and cushions as you can and, if you don't already have one, buy a large beanbag. These are all extremely useful for finding a comfortable position during labor. A hard-backed chair to sit on and lean over, or a low stool to squat over, will also be useful. It is a good idea to have someone come over to help look after your other children, so you and your partner can concentrate on your delivery.

Sustenance during labor

You might need some high-energy food to keep you going during labor and, if it is long, you may find that immediately after the birth you are ravenously hungry. Make sure your fridge and cupboards are full before your due date.

Mom-to-be

You are now in the home stretch and will find your relationship with your baby growing as you become familiar with his movements and sleep periods. It is a good idea to "test" for your baby's movements. During one hour in the morning and evening, you should see whether you can feel at least ten movements. If so, everything is fine. If not, you should not hesitate to contact your healthcare provider.

Now you will probably start to have appointments with your healthcare provider every two weeks. You may be offered a glucose screen (for diabetes) and a blood test for anemia. If you are Rh negative (see page 22), you may receive an injection of Rh immuno-globulin to prevent you from developing antibodies that can cause problems if in future you become pregnant with an Rh-positive baby.

Baby

Now at the start of his third trimester, he weighs about one-third of his estimated birth weight. He continues to make breathing movements, with the fluid entering his main air passageways and not his lungs, and the necessary muscles are developing well. Occasionally he hiccups, which you may feel.

His skin is red and now completely covered by vernix, and his head hair is longer. Subcutaneous fat deposition continues and he is now large enough to determine his presentation. This is his orientation in the womb—that is head first, or buttocks or feet first (known as breech). Rarely, a baby will be sideways.

He hears more and often sucks his thumb or fingers. If your baby is a boy, his testes have nearly completed their descent into the scrotum; if a girl, the labia are still small and don't yet cover her clitoris.

Positioning

If not already in the preferred head-down position for birth, your baby still has enough room to change his position in the next two months.

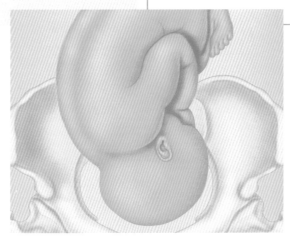

BABY'S LENGTH AND WEIGHT
His length, from crown to rump, will be nearly 10 inches and he will weigh almost 2½ pounds.

You should be seeing your healthcare provider every two weeks starting now. Be sure to sign up for childbirth education classes.

DATES FOR YOUR DIARY

MONDAY	TUESDAY	WEDNESDAY	THURSDAY	FRIDAY	SATURDAY/SUNDAY

Giving birth before your due date can be extremely worrying for parents because the risk of complications with a preterm baby is naturally higher than for a baby who is fully mature.

What is prematurity?

Any baby born at less than 37 weeks from the mother's LMP is said to be premature. In most of these cases, the baby's organs will not be sufficiently developed and her survival will depend on expert care. Premature babies generally begin life in an incubator in a neonatal intensive care unit (NICU).

What are the risks?

A premature baby is unable to maintain her body heat effectively and cannot breathe normally. She is at increased risk of neurological, heart, lung, and gastrointestinal problems, as well as being more susceptible to infection because her immune system is not ready to cope with life outside the protective uterus.

Life in an incubator

If your baby is born prematurely (or with a low birth weight), she will be placed in an incubator, which will provide vital warmth; most likely, she will be hooked up to breathing and feeding tubes and a cardiac monitor. Porthole openings in the side walls of the transparent incubator provide access for the nursing staff to care for your baby and enable you to stroke your baby until she is allowed out for you to hold and feed her. If you decide to breastfeed, your milk can be expressed and fed to her.

Physical contact

Once your baby is ready to leave her incubator, you should be encouraged to provide her with skin-to-skin contact (known as kangaroo care), which has been shown to have many benefits. It makes breastfeeding and bonding with your baby easier, and babies held this way have been shown to gain weight more readily and leave the hospital sooner.

Care once home

You will need to have a supply of smaller diapers, undershirts, and outfits, as well as a suitable car seat (there are a few models available designed for babies as small as 4½ pounds). You also may need to adjust your "nursing skills" when dispensing medications and vitamins,

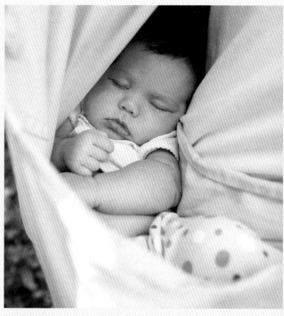

Using a sling
A premature baby thrives if freqently in close contact with her mother's body, both naked and clothed.

and be able to follow very specific instructions about feeding schedules or caring for ongoing medical conditions.

Premature infants have immature immune mechanisms, so you will need to limit holding, touching, and close contact to only a few close relatives or friends, and only after they have washed their hands thoroughly. Prohibit anyone with a contagious illness from visiting and avoid public places where people are in close proximity. You will visit your healthcare provider frequently to discuss your baby's feeding and nutrition, the status of any remaining medical problems, and her rate of growth.

There is great variation as to when "catching up" is achieved. A healthy premature infant usually will have entered the range of normal—in terms of growth and mastery of developmental skills—by a chronological age of 12 to 18 months.

Mom-to-be

You may be leaking colostrum or "early milk" from your breasts. This is a sticky, watery substance that will provide your baby's first food if you breastfeed. Colostrum precedes the proper milk supply, which may not start for one or two days after delivery. Your breasts are producing this milk under the influence of prolactin, a hormone that is now being produced in large quantities, due to stimulation by your baby.

Your uterus is getting much bigger and now exerts pressure on your internal organs, so having to urinate frequently can be a potential problem when you are away from home.

Baby

Space in the uterus is cramped but she still stretches and flexes her limbs and sometimes kicks. Her head, which is growing more hair, is more in proportion to the rest of her body as her body's weight increases. The soft and expandable bones in her skull enable her brain to develop rapidly, and brain tissue continues to grow.

Her brain is now adept at controlling bodily functions such as breathing and body temperature, but if she were born now she would still require an incubator for warmth.

Her senses are more responsive. For example, her eyes have greater sensitvity to the light and her ability to hear, taste, and smell is greater.

Becoming more rounded

Now that your baby has gained weight, she looks plumper and less wrinkled. Her ability to keep herself warm improves with the amount of body fat she lays down.

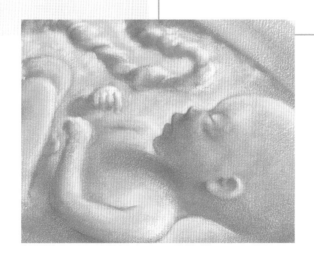

BABY'S LENGTH AND WEIGHT
Her length, from crown to rump, will be about 10¼ inches and she will weigh about 2¾ pounds.

If leaking breasts are a problem, buy some breast pads to prevent your clothes from being stained.

DATES FOR YOUR DIARY

MONDAY	TUESDAY	WEDNESDAY	THURSDAY	FRIDAY	SATURDAY/SUNDAY

PREPARING FOR LABOR

As your pregnancy advances, it is a good idea to prepare yourself for your labor. Do this by setting aside time to practice certain exercises, which will help you get into suitable birth positions (see page 71) and by making sure you know how to relax (see page 34). Starting to prepare yourself this week will be extremely helpful if your baby happens to come early.

Squatting

This position is very useful during labor because it enables the pull of gravity to help a baby along the birth canal. Squatting exercises will open your pelvis to its widest and help stretch your perineum (the area between your anus and vagina), which may prevent tearing during childbirth. Unfortunately, squatting is not a position most women adopt during their everyday activities, so it may be difficult to do at first. Practice squatting by sitting on a low stool: place your feet wide apart and lean forward, keeping your back straight.

Push your knees out wide with your elbows. Once your pelvic joints are flexible and you are comfortable with the position, try to support your body weight without the aid of the stool. You can use doorknobs, a sturdy chair, or your partner for support. If you can't keep your heels on the ground, place a rolled-up blanket or towel under them.

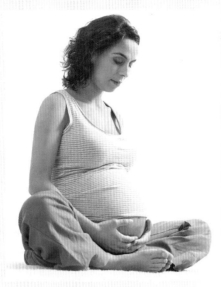

Tailor sitting
Sit with your back straight and put the soles of your feet together. Draw your heels up toward your perineum, using your arms to push down on your thighs.

Tailor sitting

This position helps strengthen the thigh muscles, which is important for holding squatting positions and improving pelvic flexibility. If you find this position difficult at first, you can use cushions under your thighs as support, or sit with your back straight against a wall. While you are in this position, concentrate on your breathing and relaxation techniques (see page 34).

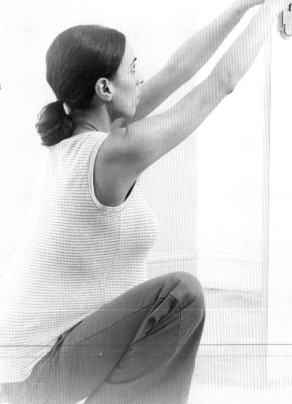

Daily squats
At first you probably won't be able to hold this squatting position for very long, but if you practice this position for a few minutes every day, then gradually you will be able to increase the length of time held.

Mom-to-be

As you become larger you are probably also becoming slower and clumsier. Remember to maintain good posture when standing and sitting (see page 32). In particular, make sure you always roll onto your side before getting up (and that you always lie on your back with your face upward and never with the front of your body facing downward) because your abdominal muscles have stretched and loosened to accommodate your growing uterus.

Getting up frequently at night to urinate may be contributing to growing fatigue, so try to get plenty of rest during the day, and going to bed early—perhaps with warmed milk (which can help you to sleep).

Baby

His lanugo is disappearing so that when he is born only a few patches may be present. His head hair is thicker and his skin less wrinkled thanks to an increase in baby fat; overall he looks a lot rounder and plumper.

His finger- and toenails are growing fast, his bone marrow has taken over red blood-cell production from the liver, and his skeleton is hardening more and more. His mimicking of breathing movements is now rhythmic as his lungs are more mature, and he still gets hiccups from swallowing amniotic fluid. Lack of space in the uterus increasingly restricts his movements, but he still kicks—often in reaction to noise. He is awake more often and his eyes open and close more frequently.

If a girl, her clitoris is prominent because the labia are still yet to cover it.

Inner activity

Your baby still has room in the uterus in which he can bring his feet up to his face. Soon, however, he won't be able to do this.

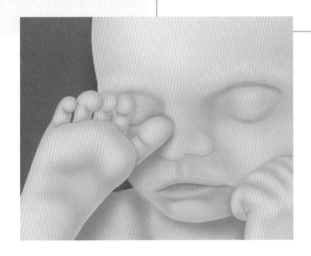

BABY'S LENGTH AND WEIGHT
His length, from crown to rump, will be around 10½ inches and he will weigh about 3 pounds.

Start finalizing your birth plan; if necessary, check with the hospital or your healthcare provider about facilities and routines.

DATES FOR YOUR DIARY

MONDAY	TUESDAY	WEDNESDAY	THURSDAY	FRIDAY	SATURDAY/SUNDAY

YOUR BIRTH PARTNER

Giving birth is a powerful emotional and physical experience, and sharing it with someone can make it that much more special. The baby's father is usually a woman's first choice for a birth partner because he will usually have been involved in the pregnancy from the beginning. However, depending on your circumstances, you may want to ask your mother, sister, close friend, or birth specialist (doula) to provide the necessary support.

Before the delivery

Ask your birth partner to attend childbirth education classes with you, so that he or she can learn about the changes you are experiencing during pregnancy and the feelings you may have during labor. It is also a good idea to practice labor exercises and breathing and relaxation techniques together, so your birth partner will be able to coach and support you confidently during labor.

If you are planning to give birth in hospital, you should take your birth partner on a tour of the facilities there so that he or she will be familiar with the surroundings. You should also name your birth partner in your birth plan (see page 32) and write down the role you would like him or her to perform while you are in labor. Your birth partner should also be introduced to your doctor or nurse-midwife, preferably before labor begins.

Discuss with your birth partner beforehand the kind of labor you envisage. It is impossible to predict just how the delivery will proceed, so it is important to be flexible and discuss all the possible options (see page 24). During the birth you may find that you are in too much pain or you don't want to break your concentration to talk. This is when your birth partner should take over and communicate your wishes to medical staff attending you.

Being together

Before the birth, your partner can share in your pregnancy and help with breathing and positional exercises. During the birth, even if you are managing well, the constant presence of a birth partner will be reassuring, helping you relax and offering you encouragement.

Birth partner help during a cesarean section

If you have a cesarean section (see page 82), in most cases your birth partner can be with you in the operating theater. He or she will stand by your head and should keep you informed of progress. You and your partner should be able to get acquainted with your baby while you are being stitched. However, if you have an emergency cesarean under a general anesthetic, your birth partner generally will not be allowed in the operating room but will be waiting for you when you wake up.

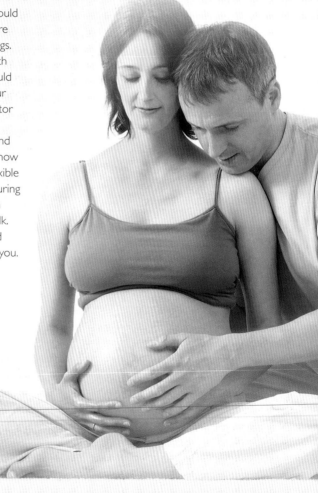

Mom-to-be

Backaches may continue to be a problem as the ligaments and muscles supporting the small of your back relax and loosen in preparation for the rigors of labor. Because your balance is also affected, you should be extra careful when climbing stairs, walking on uneven surfaces, and when out in wet or icy weather conditions.

The average weight gain for a woman at this point in a singleton pregnancy is 19 pounds. This gain is made up of the baby, the placenta, amniotic fluid, enlarged breasts and uterus, an increase in blood volume, and stored fat, protein, and water.

You should be thinking about baby's name—and maybe choosing announcements.

Baby

If your baby were born now, her chances of survival have improved this week, because her lungs are better able to inflate properly. This is because there is now more (though not sufficient) protective surfactant.

Weight gain and brain growth continue, and she is almost fully mature except for her lungs and digestive tract. Her eyes are pigmented, though their final color won't be established until she is six to nine months old. Her eyelids are open during active times and closed during sleep, as they will be in real life.

A little more than 15 fluid ounces of your blood flows through the uterine wall, and her blood vessels are coming into very close contact with the capillaries of the placenta that carry her blood. Although the two bloods never mix, they are separated only by a very thin wall—the placental barrier—across which water, nutrients, and waste are exchanged.

Vital secretions

Your baby's lungs are producing more surfactant. This substance prevents the air sacs from sticking together or collapsing when outside the uterus, enabling her to take in air and breathe properly once born.

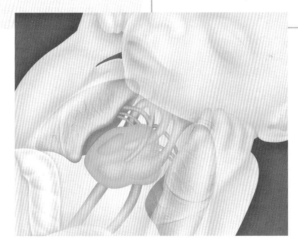

BABY'S LENGTH AND WEIGHT
Her length, from crown to rump, will be around 11 inches and she will weigh about 3½ pounds.

At your appointments, your blood pressure will be more closely monitored, since a rise in pressure can be a sign of preeclampsia.

DATES FOR YOUR DIARY

MONDAY	TUESDAY	WEDNESDAY	THURSDAY	FRIDAY	SATURDAY/SUNDAY

BONDING

You may well be one of those women who immediately falls in love with her baby. But if your emotions don't overflow at first sight, you needn't worry—research has indicated that bonding is not usually an instantaneous process. In fact, most women take time to develop a special, intimate relationship with their baby, especially if the birth was difficult.

Bonding
Most experts believe that in order to facilitate the bonding process, you should spend time cuddling your baby as soon as he is born. Having just emerged from the comfort of your uterus, your baby will most likely be feeling very unsettled, insecure, and vulnerable. Skin-to-skin contact will reassure a newborn and will help you get to know your baby.

The more in touch you are with him, the more your feelings will grow, and the happier and healthier your baby will become. This is why it is very important for you to be involved in your baby's care, even while you are in the hospital. If your baby has problems and is taken to a neonatal intensive care unit, you should make an effort to visit him frequently. The sight of your baby in an incubator hooked up to various drips may be distressing for you, but your baby will appreciate the comfort you can provide if you gently stroke him with your fingers, as soon as you are allowed, and softly talk or sing to him.

A father's love
Bonding is not limited to mother and baby: your partner should be involved too. Most hospital staff will give you both time alone immediately after the birth to get to know your baby. If this is not hospital policy, you might like to request this in your birth plan. Fathers often have extended visiting hours, so ensure your partner takes full advantage of these. If your baby is in the neonatal intensive care unit, dad should visit frequently, so your baby maintains contact with both parents. Encourage dad to cradle, bathe, and change your baby's diapers as often as possible. Your baby will soon recognize his smell and voice, which is so crucial to the bonding process.

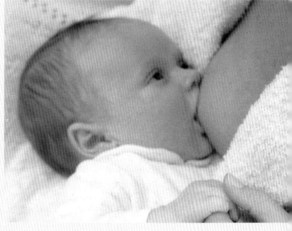

A moment to cherish
Spending time with your baby, breastfeeding or otherwise, will stir powerful maternal feelings and facilitates bonding.

Breastfeeding
This natural process is an ideal way to convey love, as well as sustenance, to your newborn. In addition to nutrients, breast milk supplies antibodies vital for a baby's health, so breastfeeding as soon as possible is desirable. Very few women are incapable of breastfeeding (surgery or disease, however, may affect the necessary underlying structures). A woman's ability to produce milk is not affected by breast size or nipple shape, because a baby sucks from the whole areola and not just the nipple. Moreover, a baby is born with built-in reflexes that ensure she can locate, latch onto, and suck from a breast. However, some mothers may need help with technique to be completely successful. If you have problems, seek the advice of a lactation consultant or a breastfeeding organization, such as La Leche League, or other online sources. Your healthcare provider should be able to point you in the right direction. The sooner you seek help, the more likely you will master the process.

Mom-to-be

This week your growing uterus may trigger a new problem: your baby is probably head-down by now and large enough that his legs reach up to your ribs. The pressure on them can make your ribcage sore, especially if your baby's feet get caught. Avoid this uncomfortable situation by sitting up straight as often as possible.

Your internal organs can become a little displaced, but this is not normally a cause for concern. Fluid retention, however, may be an issue. It can result in varicose veins and swollen ankles and fingers. Remove any rings from your fingers if they become tight, and don't wear restrictive clothing.

Continue taking your prenatal supplements because your baby's demand for vitamins and minerals is especially high just now.

Stay positive! There are only eight weeks to go until you meet your wonderful new baby.

Baby

All his senses are complete and in working order, while his limbs and body continue to fill out. His body is now in proportion to his head size. His head hair and toenails continue to grow.

His lungs and digestive tract continue to mature and he practices breathing, which strengthens and develops his lungs. He is passing urine efficiently from his bladder.

By now his head should be down in your uterus, pressing against your pelvic floor, in preparation for birth, which can leave him free to kick at your ribcage.

He sleeps about 90 to 95 percent of the day (and is probably dreaming), his eyeballs moving behind closed lids.

If a boy, his testes have descended and both testicles are in his scrotum.

Almost ready

Your baby now looks just as he will when born: his face and body have filled out and all his facial features are developed. His eyes are open more of the time.

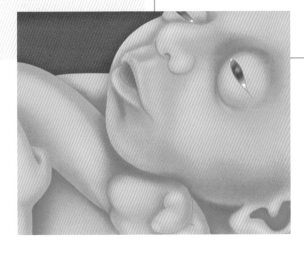

BABY'S LENGTH AND WEIGHT
His length, from crown to rump, will be around 11½ inches and he will weigh about 4 pounds.

You may be starting your childbirth education classes this week.

DATES FOR YOUR DIARY

MONDAY	TUESDAY	WEDNESDAY	THURSDAY	FRIDAY	SATURDAY/SUNDAY

PACKING FOR THE HOSPITAL

It is a good idea to prepare all the things you will need for your stay in the hospital about a month in advance of your estimated date of delivery. If you go into labor unexpectedly, you will not have time to gather all the things you need and this lack of preparedness can cause added stress. Pack all your items in a large overnight bag and store it in a place well known to you and your birth partner. You should also make some contingency plans in the event that you go into labor when you are away from home. If this is the case, your birth partner (if it is not your live-in partner) needs a spare key to your home to get in and pick up your hospital bag for you.

If you have a cesarean section, you will be in the hospital for longer; in this case, your partner may be able to bring going-home clothes for you and your baby at a later date.

For your baby

Check with your hospital whether you need to bring baby supplies, other than a going-home outfit and an infant car seat. Usually the hospital will provide diapers and some formula milk, if you are not breastfeeding.

Useful but nonessential items include a cell phone (with charger), camera (with spare batteries or charger), reading material, snacks, and money for vending machines and parking.

Comfort aids

Your birth partner can use the following to help you relax while you are in labor: pregnancy-safe aromatherapy oils; hot and cold packs or lotions; and wooden rolling balls (or tennis balls) for massaging your back and shoulders. Sucking on ice can help relieve pain, so check whether there is an ice-dispensing machine near your room.

IN THE BAG

- Copy of your birth plan
- Dressing gown, nightdress, and underwear
- Warm socks
- Breastfeeding supplies: nursing bra and breast pads
- Thick-absorbency sanitary towels
- Toiletries, makeup, and hairbrush
- Toothbrush and toothpaste
- Loose clothes and comfortable shoes
- Going-home clothes for baby: undershirt, babygrow or onesie, hat, and shawl
- Extra bag for taking home gifts and supplies

Mom-to-be

The volume of your uterus has grown 500 times over the course of your pregnancy and amniotic fluid is at its highest level. Physiological anemia (see page 49) starts to fade as red blood cell production catches up with that of plasma. You may also experience strangely vivid dreams and feel a more frequent need to urinate. If your baby has assumed a head-down position, you may find it easier to breathe and any indigestion should start to improve.

Baby

Restricted inside your cramped uterus, she still sleeps a lot of the time, dreaming vividly. When she is awake she is quietly alert: listening, feeling, maybe even seeing dim shapes, but, above all, learning, as the billions of neurons in her brain forge literally trillions of connections. She is active, though by now her movements are curtailed to a few strong kicks and jabs.

Her bones are fully developed but soft; she is storing iron, calcium, and phosphorous to use in further bone development. The mechanism for controlling body temperature, the hypothalamus, starts to function in her brain, but if born now she would still need to be in an incubator to stay warm enough and although she makes rhythmic breathing movements, her lungs are still immature and she would struggle to breathe air.

Now fatter with pinker skin, your baby should have settled into her birth position and the doctor or nurse-midwife (and you) can probably tell which way she is presenting.

Recognizable behavior

Your baby will increasingly make more of the gestures of a full-term infant. She can stick out her tongue (perhaps tasting the amniotic fluid), yawn, grimace, and in some cases, appear to smile.

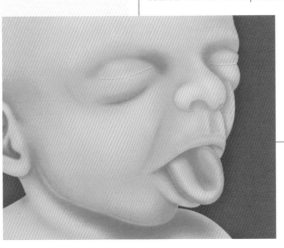

BABY'S LENGTH AND WEIGHT
Her length, from crown to rump, will be almost 12 inches and she will weigh almost 4½ pounds.

Make sure you check on your baby's movements each day; ask your healthcare provider what to look for.

DATES FOR YOUR DIARY

MONDAY	TUESDAY	WEDNESDAY	THURSDAY	FRIDAY	SATURDAY/SUNDAY

LABOR POSITIONS

When the time comes, your body will probably let you know the best positions for birth. In the past, women were made to stay on their backs with their feet up, which is actually very uncomfortable and fights against the pull of gravity. Some women now choose to be propped up in sitting positions on their hospital beds with their legs wide apart, while others want to move around, squat on the floor, or stand upright supported by their partner.

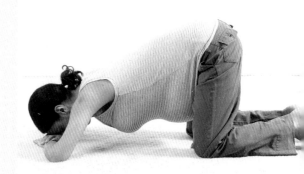

During the first stage

While your cervix is dilating and effacing, you will be experiencing contractions of increasing intensity and frequency. During each contraction, lean against your partner or a wall or over a chair. You can also kneel on all fours, in which case it is a good idea to have something cushioning your knees. Between contractions, try standing up, walking or, supported by your birth partner, rocking your pelvis from side to side.

All fours position

This relieves an aching back by pushing your uterus forward to take pressure off of your spine. Also try rocking your hips from side to side.

Side lying

This position is good if you have an epidural or when you get tired because it can make contractions more effective and help slow down the baby's descent if he's coming too quickly.

During delivery

Give your baby as much room as possible by widening your knees and allowing your uterus to tilt forward. Like most women, you may not be able to hold a squat position for long periods, so drape an arm around your birth partner and nurse-midwife for support. A variation of this is to kneel down, supported on the bed or floor.

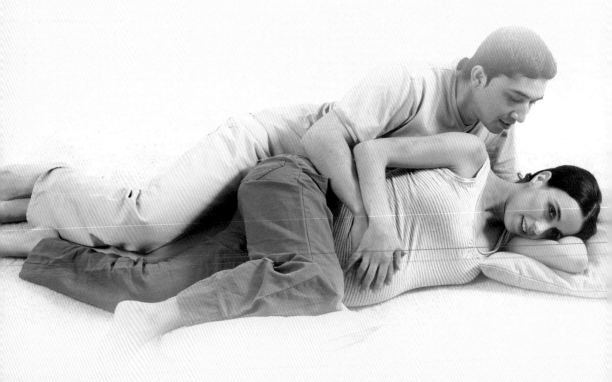

Mom-to-be

Braxton Hicks contractions (see page 51) have probably become more frequent—they feel like a tightening at the top of the uterus that spreads down and then relaxes. The difference between Braxton Hicks contractions and real labor contractions is that real labor contractions become progressively longer in duration, more painful, and do not go away. If your waters break, call your healthcare provider immediately.

Your weight gain begins to slow, but you may be surprised at how big your tummy has grown.

Baby

The hair on his head continues to thicken. At the same time he is shedding almost all of his lanugo, although the vernix is still thick. His skin is less wrinkled and is getting pinker. His tiny, sharp fingernails reach the tips of his fingers.

His adrenal glands, which are producing ten times more steroid hormone (a substance like androgen that indirectly stimulates lactation) than a normal adult, are the same size as those of an adolescent. These glands shrink after birth. His bones are hardening, except for those in his skull, which remain flexible to enable him to traverse the birth canal more easily.

His immune system can fight mild infections now, except for his lungs, which may still need time to develop. He is developing quickly so, if you gave birth now, he would probably have nearly the same long-term outcome as a full-term baby.

Space is becoming restricted in the uterus, so his movements become fewer but more powerful and sustained.

Preparation for feeding

Although thumbsucking isn't yet connected with satisfying hunger, your baby will practice it because it is a way of exploring things. Once born, he will use his sucking reflex to find food.

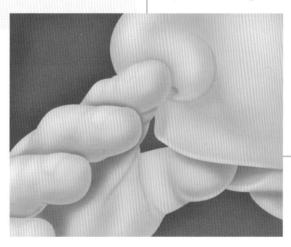

BABY'S LENGTH AND WEIGHT
His length, from crown to rump, will be around 12½ inches and he will weigh about 5 pounds.

 If you haven't already, you should start your childbirth education classes now.

DATES FOR YOUR DIARY

MONDAY	TUESDAY	WEDNESDAY	THURSDAY	FRIDAY	SATURDAY/SUNDAY

PAIN RELIEF DURING LABOR

All women use one or more pain-relieving strategies during labor. Some prefer natural forms of pain relief—relaxation and breathing techniques, changes in position, water, acupuncture, or hypnosis—but most will use a drug. Sometimes fear or anxiety will increase pain sensations, which is why it is important to be aware of the process your body will go through during labor.

Find out your hospital's policy on pain relief and discuss the options with your healthcare provider. You may decide you don't want pain relief, but you won't really know how it feels until you start going into labor.

Analgesics and anesthetics

There are two types of pain-relieving drugs—analgesics and anesthetics. Analgesics relieve pain without total loss of feeling or muscle movement. They are used to lessen pain but usually do not stop you from feeling pain completely. Anesthetics block all feeling, including pain.

Systemic analgesics act on the whole nervous system, rather than a specific area, to lessen pain. They will not cause you to lose consciousness, and are often administered, usually as a shot into a muscle or vein, during early labor to allow you to rest. Local anesthesia affects only a small part of the body to provide relief from the pain in that part. Such drugs are injected into the area around the nerves that carry feeling to the vagina, vulva, and perineum and are given just before delivery. They also are used when an episiotomy is needed or when any vaginal tears that happened during birth are repaired.

Regional analgesia and regional anesthesia

These act on a specific region of the body and can lessen or block pain below the waist. They include the epidural block (the most common type of pain relief administered in labor in the US), spinal block, and combined spinal-epidural (CSE) block.

Epidural block

This anesthetic injection numbs the lower half of your body, so will need to follow instructions on when to push and pant. After a local anesthetic is given to freeze the back, a fine tube is inserted between your vertebrae into the spinal cord, and the epidural is administered through it. The tube is taped in place in case you need a refill. It takes about 20 minutes to administer and the effects last throughout your labor since the anesthetist can continue to give you medication when you need it.

Help with pain

Your birth partner can provide comfort and encouragement but an anesthetist is required to carry out an epidural and to top it off as needed.

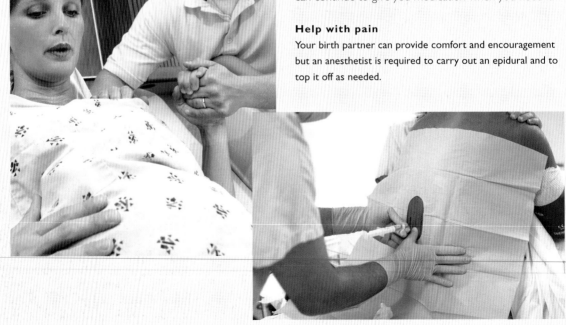

Mom-to-be

You probably feel cramped and heavy, and as though you don't have room to breathe, or to take in food. Try to eat small meals at frequent intervals, get plenty of rest, and to avoid swollen ankles and immobility, don't sit or stand in one position for too long. If you are making long car journeys, take regular breaks to get out and walk around.

You should be preparing for your leave of absence from work now if you haven't already done so. Other preparations you need to make include buying some properly fitted nursing bras and attending childbirth education classes.

Baby

Fat deposition continues, especially around your baby's shoulders, which are becoming plump and chubby, and there is hardly any room now for her to move around. Babies often have facial scratch marks at birth from the time when their arms were held close to their face.

Her central nervous system is maturing and she stays awake and aware for longer periods of time. Her digestive system is nearly complete and her lungs nearly fully mature.

She is still shedding her lanugo, although there may still be some present by the time she is born. Her eyes are blue but this may well change after birth.

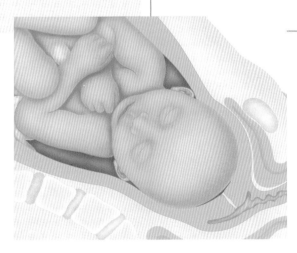

Positioned for birth
The baby is low down in the uterus, her head near the cervix and her limbs tightly compressed. When contractions start, her head will push against the surface to thin it out, so opening out the birth canal.

BABY'S LENGTH AND WEIGHT
Her length, from crown to rump, will be around 13 inches and she will weigh about 5½ pounds.

Get your partner make a practice run to the hospital so he/she knows where to avoid traffic jams and other problems.

DATES FOR YOUR DIARY

MONDAY	TUESDAY	WEDNESDAY	THURSDAY	FRIDAY	SATURDAY/SUNDAY

If your labor is induced or it is deemed high risk, or as a routine labor practice in some hospitals, electronic fetal monitoring will be used to continuously check your baby's heartbeat. You may like to discuss the alternatives with your healthcare provider.

Induction of labor

Labor may be started artificially if your baby is at risk because you are suffering from preeclampsia or diabetes, or your placenta is not supplying him with adequate nutrients or you are overdue (see page 86). There are various methods.

Oxytocin

This is a hormone produced naturally by your body, which causes your uterus to contract. You may be given a synthetic form in an intravenous drip. (Pitocin and Syntocinon are brand names for these drugs.) This can cause contractions to come suddenly and more severely than usual, so if you are given oxytocin to induce labor, you may also need additional pain relief (see page 74).

Keeping check

Many women find the visible signs of their unborn baby's stable heartbeat reassuring. However, the printouts need to be interpreted carefully, so make sure your healthcare provider explains them to you thoroughly.

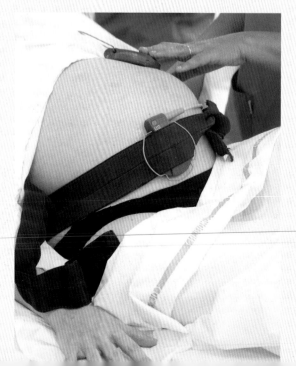

Prostaglandin suppositories and gels

These are inserted high into the vagina and will soften your cervix so that it starts to thin (efface) and widen (dilate), allowing the first stage of labor to proceed. Prostaglandin suppositories will also stimulate your own natural production of prostaglandin, which causes your uterus to contract. Suppositories and gels are very safe and your movements are not restricted after the first 30 minutes or so. This means you can walk around while you have one inserted, which can also help bring on labor.

Artificial rupturing of the membranes (AROM)

This is also called an amniotomy. A small plastic tool with a crochet-like hook at the end, is inserted through your vagina into your cervix. The hook ruptures the amniotic sac releasing the water inside. Once your waters break, the pressure within your uterus changes. Your baby's head drops into your pelvis and puts direct pressure onto the cervix, which can help start labor. If AROM does not induce labor, you may need medication to start contractions; now that your baby is not encased in the amniotic sac, he is at risk of infections entering through your cervix.

Fetal monitoring

In the early stages of labor, you will be fitted with two transducers—one of which has an ultrasound device that picks up the baby's heartbeat and the other a pressure-sensoring device, which picks up the strength and duration of each contraction. The transducers are attached by wires to a machine that records the baby's heartbeat and your contractions on a continual printout.

During the later stages, your caregiver may also monitor your baby's heartbeat by placing a Doppler fetal-monitor probe up against your abdomen, through which can be heard your baby's heartbeat.

If you are a high-risk case, a small electrode on a wire will be threaded through your vagina and cervix to be attached to your baby's head (or buttocks if he is breech). The wire is connected to a monitor and secured by tape to your inner thigh. The electrode picks up your baby's heartbeat and this again is recorded on a computer printout.

Mom-to-be

The top of your uterus now reaches its highest point, just below your breastbone, so breathing may be uncomfortable and you may get jabbing pains in your ribcage. Your childbirth education classes are in full swing and you're probably seeing your healthcare provider weekly. In fact, your whole life is gearing up for the birth. If you feel a bit overwhelmed by it all, remember that it's your pregnancy and you are in charge. You set the agenda for your delivery with a birth plan (see pages 92 and 93), and you decide what sort of pain relief you plan to use (see page 74).

One unfortunate side effect of pregnancy hormones is the synchronization of your hair follicles. Normally your hairs grow at different rates and so fall out at different times. Now a lot of them will fall out together, probably just after the birth. Don't worry about this, though, because they will grow back soon!

Baby

He continues to gain weight and has almost reached his birth length, making space in the uterus severely restricted. While he cannot wriggle much, his kicks are forceful. You may be able to see the outline of a certain body part such as an elbow or heel appearing under your skin.

His skull is firm but not hard, with enough flexibility for it to deform slightly when he is squeezing down the birth canal; he may engage this week or next (see page 78). His kidneys are completely developed and his liver can process some waste. His digestive system and lungs are fully mature; when he breathes, he is able to produce the protective surfactant.

He is awake for longer periods and his range of facial expressions is greater.

Baby face
Your baby has characteristically plump, full baby cheeks, due to a combination of fat deposits and powerful sucking muscles, perhaps honed by several months of sucking his thumb.

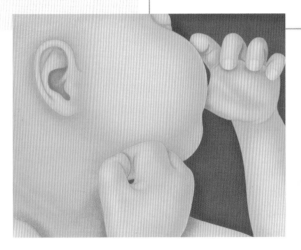

BABY'S LENGTH AND WEIGHT
His length, from crown to rump, will be around 13½ inches and he will weigh about 6 pounds.

Your birth partner and healthcare provider should be given a copy of your birth plan by this week.

DATES FOR YOUR DIARY

MONDAY	TUESDAY	WEDNESDAY	THURSDAY	FRIDAY	SATURDAY/SUNDAY

RECOGNIZING LABOR

The exact cause of the onset of labor remains unknown. The most widely held theory is that the baby produces substances that result in a change in pregnancy hormones. But you will know you are in labor when you experience regular contractions. Prior to that, there will be a few other signs that labor is near.

Engagement

Between two and four weeks before labor starts, the baby's head will descend lower into your pelvis. This is known as engagement, and there are some related benefits and minor discomforts to a baby's head being lower down. While you'll have more space to breathe, you will also pass water and have bowel movements more frequently, have aches in your pubic bones and back, sharp twinges in your pelvis, and have swollen legs and feet. Pelvic tilts (see page 30) and lying on your left side can help to relieve some of this pelvic pressure.

Nesting instinct

During the last month, you'll find you have a sudden desire to empty drawers, clear out cupboards, and scrub your home from top to bottom. This is a built-in maternal urge to prepare the home for the imminent arrival of the baby. While you want to make the most of this burst of energy, try not to overdo it.

Mucus plug and bloodstained show

As the cervix softens, shortens, and begins to dilate, the mucus plug that has sealed the cervix for most of your pregnancy will be dislodged and a small amount of bright red or brownish mucus known as a "bloodstained show" usually appears. A show may also appear as a heavier discharge or it may be unnoticeable. If you have a show, contact your healthcare provider for advice.

Rupture of membranes

The amniotic sac containing the fluid around the baby will usually rupture—known as the "waters breaking"—at some point during labor. Occasionally, however, it may rupture before contractions begin in earnest. If your waters break at home, you need to make a note of the time they break and the consistency (fluid containing meconium would be dangerous), and notify your healthcare provider.

Amniotic fluid is usually clear and odorless, and once the bag of waters has ruptured at term, it will go on leaking until delivery (urine or vaginal secretions may leak from time to time). If you become aware of something pulsing in your vagina after your waters break, this may be a prolapsed cord. Seek medical help urgently.

Contractions

At some point, any brief, irregular contractions will be replaced by ones that have a rhythmic pattern and longer length. These contractions progressively contract the upper uterus while stretching the lower part and opening or dilating the cervix. By this mechanism, the powerful upper uterine muscles push your baby through the stretchable lower uterus. Sometimes contractions are felt strongly in the back. If you experience back pain every 5 minutes, call your healthcare provider and get to the hospital.

When to go to the hospital

The early part of labor—with cramps, a backache, increased urination, bowel movements, and vaginal discharge, pelvic pressure, and leg and hip cramps—can take hours. If you are able to manage the discomfort, stay at home in familiar surroundings. If the contractions first appear at night, try to continue resting as much as possible. You should leave for the hospital when you can no longer ignore the discomfort and contractions are so intense that you are unable to hold a conversation during one, or if the contractions have been regular for more than an hour—five minutes apart, each lasting between 45 and 60 seconds. Intense contractions that are less than three minutes apart are often a signal that birth is very near.

Mom-to-be

This week or possibly later if this isn't your first pregnancy, your baby should engage. Her head (assuming she is a cephalic presentation, see page 80) will drop down into your pelvis. You will feel this dropping sensation as an easing of pressure on your ribs and internal organs. Breathing and eating should become easier. Your uterus is now pressing down hard on your bladder, however, so expect even more frequent urges to urinate. If this is your first pregnancy, it is likely to go to full term, but if you have had children before, and particularly if you are expecting twins, you can expect to deliver sooner. The average length of pregnancy for twins is 37 weeks, so be prepared by filling the tank of your car with gas and ensuring that your partner is contactable at all times.

Baby

She could now be born at any time. However, this does not mean that she has stopped growing or developing; fat continues to be laid down at the rate of more than ½ ounce per day, and myelination (the protective coating) of the neurons in the brain is still in progress (it will continue after birth). She may even grow a little in length this week.

Her immune system continues to develop to protect her once she's born. Antibodies she doesn't produce herself she'll receive from you via the placenta, to give her a temporary boost in immunity for the first few 3 months of life (see page 83).

She still spends most of her time asleep, but when she's awake, her eyes and limbs will move constantly, as much as they can in an increasingly restricted space.

Most of her lanugo has disappeared but her head hair is up to 1 inch in length.

Cramped quarters
Research suggests that a baby triggers labor by producing the necessary hormones in response to being in a restrictive environment.

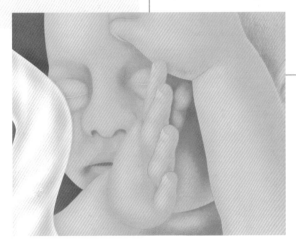

BABY'S LENGTH AND WEIGHT
Her length, from crown to rump, will be almost 14 inches and she will weigh about 6½ pounds.

If you are expecting twins, be prepared. The birth can happen or be scheduled for this week.

DATES FOR YOUR DIARY

MONDAY	TUESDAY	WEDNESDAY	THURSDAY	FRIDAY	SATURDAY/SUNDAY

SPECIAL DELIVERIES

If your baby is in a breech position or you are expecting twins, your delivery will usually need additional medical assistance. More often than not this means giving birth by cesarean section but, depending on your situation, it may still be possible to have a vaginal delivery.

Breech delivery

Toward the end of labor, most babies will be lying with their head facing the cervix. The medical term for this is vertex or cephalic presentation. Some babies, however, are in upright positions and will stay that way until the birth. Breech delivery—when a baby is born buttocks or feet first—occurs about three times in every hundred deliveries. Sometimes a doctor or nurse-midwife may try to turn a baby around by gently exerting pressure on the mother's abdomen while she is lying down. This is called external cephalic version (ECV) and is successful about 50 percent of the time.

Breech babies can be born vaginally, but need to be carefully assisted by medical staff. If there is not enough space in your pelvis, the umbilical cord may become compressed while your baby's head is being born, thereby cutting off his oxygen supply. Also, your baby's

buttocks may not stretch the cervix sufficiently for his head to be born—the head being the largest part of a newborn. This may result in forceps being required to deliver the head. Occasionally, a ventouse (vacuum extractor) will be used. Instead of metal tongs, a soft cup is placed on the baby's head and suction helps to pull the baby out.

Breech births, with or without forceps or a ventouse, will necessitate an episiotomy because baby's buttocks won't have stretched your perineum sufficiently. This involves the doctor making a small incision through the perineum to enlarge the vagina. This is done both to accommodate any use of forceps and to prevent tears occurring, which can prove more difficult to heal.

Twin delivery

Sometimes, in a twin pregnancy, the uterus is stretched so widely that labor can start a few weeks before your due date. Quite often, the first baby will be born head first and the second will be a breech delivery. If one or both babies are breech, your doctor may recommend that you have a cesarean section. In some cases, the first, usually larger baby, is delivered vaginally and the second, generally smaller baby, by cesarean. There is usually a five- to 10-minute gap between each birth. Because there is a greater chance of complications with multiple births, if you are expecting twins, you are quite likely to have continual fetal monitoring throughout your labor and delivery. You also will probably be given an epidural for pain relief, which is will be useful if an emergency cesarean is required.

Assisted delivery

If the mother is having difficulty pushing, or the baby needs to be turned or born quickly, forceps may be used to assist delivery. An episiotomy will be done if forceps are used.

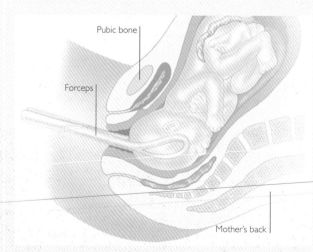

Pubic bone

Forceps

Mother's back

Mom-to-be

Just before your real contractions begin you may experience false labor contractions. Not to be confused with Braxton Hicks contractions (see page 51), these may be nearly as strong as the real thing, but do not become regular and disappear if you move around. How can you tell the difference? If you're not sure, it is unlikely to be the real thing.

Some women may experience a depressed mood, the result of a mixture of anxiety about the birth, fatigue due to a lack of sleep, and a desire for the pregnancy to end. If you feel this way, speak to your healthcare provider and try to focus on the thought that your baby soon will be here.

Baby

Now clinically mature, he is ready to be born. Over the last few weeks your baby has been building up greenish-black waste material, called meconium, in his intestines. It is primarily made up of the products of blood cell breakdown, cells shed by his intestinal lining, and skin cells and lanugo, which have passed into the amniotic fluid and been swallowed. Meconium will be the first waste your baby passes after birth; occasionally it gets excreted before delivery, and the baby arrives covered in unpleasant waste.

The placenta begins to age now because its role in sustaining your baby comes to an end. It becomes less efficient at transferring nutrients, and blood clots and calcified patches begin to show on ultrasound scans.

Your baby demonstrates a range of facial expressions in reaction to sound, touch, and other sensations. Nearly all of his lanugo hair is gone and he is being squeezed by early uterine contractions.

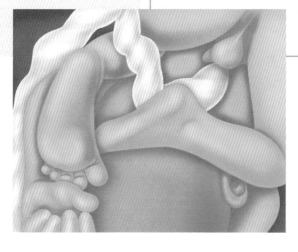

Testicular descent
If your baby is a boy, his testes should now be in his scrotum. By the time he is born, both should be in place.

BABY'S LENGTH AND WEIGHT
His length, from crown to rump, will be around 14½ to 15 inches and he will weigh about 6¾ pounds.

If your baby is in a breech position, your doctor or nurse-midwife may try turning him with external cephalic version.

DATES FOR YOUR DIARY

MONDAY	TUESDAY	WEDNESDAY	THURSDAY	FRIDAY	SATURDAY/SUNDAY

CESAREAN SECTION

According to US National Vital Statistics Report's final birth data for 2013, 32.7 percent of all births in the US were by cesarean section. Also known as a C-section, it is a very safe procedure for both mother and baby.

Reasons for a cesarean section

If your pelvis is an unusual shape or disproportionate to the size of your baby's head, your baby will be delivered by cesarean section. Other reasons for a cesarean include a twin pregnancy, placenta previa, a diabetic mother, or a large baby, or one in a breech or transverse position. Sometimes, if your labor is not progressing well or your baby has an abnormal heartbeat, an emergency cesarean will be performed to deliver the baby quickly.

Procedure

Your abdomen will be covered with antiseptic to kill off any bacteria and some pubic hair may be shaved. You will be given an epidural or spinal anesthetic (sometimes a general anesthetic is administered) and an intravenous drip; a catheter will be inserted into your bladder to

Screened off

If you are conscious throughout the procedure, you will be screened from the actual delivery. Your baby will be handed to you after initial birth checks have been made.

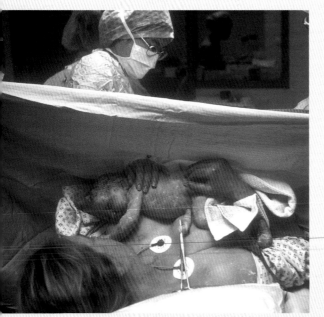

The incisions

During a cesarean, two incisions are made—one through the skin and the other through the uterine wall. The cut visible on the outside may not necessarily be in the same position as the internal incision. The cut made in your abdomen usually is just large

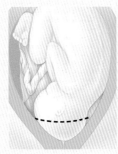

enough for your baby to be taken out. The most common is the transverse incision: a horizontal cut made across the lower part of the uterus.

empty it. A screen will be placed across your upper body so that you cannot see the operation, but an epidural means you will be conscious to receive your newborn baby, and your partner will probably be allowed to be at your side. The surgeon will make an incision in your abdominal wall and then through your uterus. He or she will then reach in and gently lift out your baby. After an initial examination, your baby will probably be handed to you. He may be slow to respond to his new environment because there has been no period of adjustment the way there would have been if he had traveled through the vaginal canal.

Meanwhile, the placenta will be removed and examined and your incision will be stitched up. The procedure takes about 30 to 60 minutes, but the delivery itself takes only five to 10 minutes.

Recovery

Because a cesarean section is major surgery, it takes a few weeks for full recovery. You will be required to stay in the hospital for a couple of days after the surgery—perhaps longer depending on your progress. It may be difficult to sit and stand straight and will hurt when you cough or laugh. Postpartum exercises are necessary to get your abdominal muscles back into shape, but your healthcare provider will advise you on this. To make breastfeeding more comfortable, lie on your side with your baby next to you.

Mom-to-be

Your cervix is ripening in preparation, and your bladder is under more pressure than ever. You're probably nervous about recognizing the onset of labor. Strong contractions that get worse when you move around and become more regular and frequent are the most reliable signs. Other indications include your waters breaking as the amniotic membrane ruptures and a show of blood as the mucus that plugged your cervical canal is dislodged (in both instances you should contact your healthcare provider immediately). However, neither of these may happen until well into the first stage of labor.

Baby

Hardly any lanugo will now remain, except perhaps on her shoulders and in the creases of her chubby body. Her toenails reach the end of her toes. The umbilical cord is about ¾ inch thick and about as long as she is, and may be knotted or wrapped around her; it is still supplying her with a lot of nutrients as she continues to gain weight.

A few of your antibodies now cross the placental barrier and enter her bloodstream, giving her immune system a temporary boost to help until it gets into full swing. These will disappear within six months.

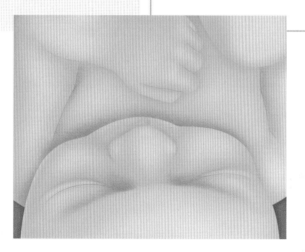

Head-down position

Your baby is almost ready to be born so you could deliver any day now. Space is very limited; the baby's limbs are pressed close against her head and trunk and her head is right up against your cervix. This pressure on your cervix will thin the tissues, creating an opening to the birth canal.

BABY'S LENGTH AND WEIGHT
Her length, from crown to rump, will be around 14½ to 15 inches and she will weigh about 7 pounds.

Time to get the groceries to make sure the fridge and cupboards are fully stocked for when you're back home with baby.

DATES FOR YOUR DIARY

MONDAY	TUESDAY	WEDNESDAY	THURSDAY	FRIDAY	SATURDAY/SUNDAY

GIVING BIRTH

There are three stages of birth. The first is when contractions start coming at regular intervals, thinning and stretching your cervix. The second is when you feel the urge to "bear down" and push your baby through the vaginal canal until she is delivered. The final stage is when the placenta detaches itself from the uterine wall and is expelled.

Transition

This marks the end of the first stage and the beginning of the second. Contractions should now last 60 to 90 seconds and occur at two- to five-minute intervals. Transition is usually the most intense physical and emotional stage of birth. Your doctor or nurse-midwife will perform a vaginal examination to check that your cervix is fully dilated (measuring approximately 4 inches) before you start pushing.

Crowning

After transition, you will probably be overwhelmed by the desire to push, and this "bearing down" is a completely involuntary action. As your baby's head reaches the end of the vaginal canal it will bulge against the perineum, causing some pain and possible bruising. It will also put pressure on your rectum, which can result in involuntary bowel movements. During each contraction your baby's head will start to show through the vagina and then recede once the contractions subside. After a few more pushes it will stay there. This is what is known as "crowning."

Being born

Once your baby's head has crowned, it will only be a matter of minutes before he is finally delivered. At this stage, you should stop pushing and start panting. This will allow your perineum to stretch and prevent tearing. Now at each contraction, your baby's head will come farther out until it appears fully outside the vagina. Once his head is out, your baby will immediately turn toward the inside of your thigh and the next contraction will probably deliver his shoulders. The rest of his body will immediately slither out, accompanied by a great gush of amniotic fluid.

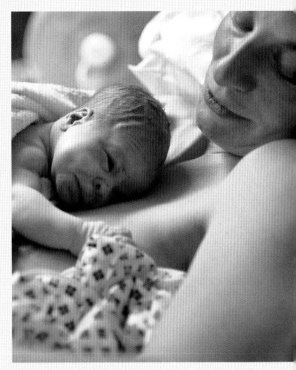

Mother and newborn
If you request that your baby be handed to you immediately after birth, you may notice that his head is slightly misshapen and that his skin may be unnaturally pale or purplish.

Delivery of the placenta

This can take up to half an hour to be expelled. You may be given Syntocinon, a synthetic oxytocin, which will help your uterus to contract and help reduce blood loss. The placenta is generally delivered with the side attached to the umbilical cord appearing first. It will be checked to see that it is complete and that no placental material remains in your uterus.

Mom-to-be

Try to stay calm while you're waiting for labor to start, and use any false or early labor contractions to practice your relaxation and breathing techniques. Once you go into full labor, it's up to your birth partner to ensure your birth plan is followed (see page 93) but you should be prepared to be flexible, because your labor is unlikely to go exactly according to plan. Be prepared also for labor to be painful. You may have already decided not to use pain relief (see page 74), but you are entitled to change your mind at almost any stage.

Baby

The look of a newborn baby is often a surprise for his parents. Firstly, his head may be misshapen, although this rapidly corrects itself within a day or two. Secondly, he may be blue, purplish, or pale yellow and he will probably be covered with a variety of substances, including waxy vernix, maternal blood, any remaining lanugo, and even some meconium if he has passed his first waste in utero. Thirdly, high hormone levels mean that his genitals may be swollen or his breasts might leak a white substance. Lastly, he may have a variety of skin discolorations, spots, and dry patches, most of which will eventually fade.

Happy landings

Once the top of your baby's head appears at the entrance to the birth canal, the rest of his head and soon his body will emerge. Changes take place inside his lungs that enable him to breathe outside the womb.

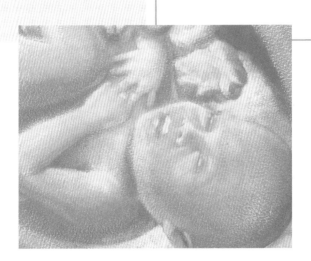

BABY'S LENGTH AND WEIGHT
His length, from crown to rump, will be about 15 inches (total length 19 inches) and he will weigh about 7 pounds.

Your baby's size and position will be assessed this week because he is due to be born.

DATES FOR YOUR DIARY

MONDAY	TUESDAY	WEDNESDAY	THURSDAY	FRIDAY	SATURDAY/SUNDAY

GOING OVERDUE

Pregnancy normally lasts 40 weeks, but you should expect your baby any time within two weeks on either side of your due date. Your pregnancy will only be officially overdue if it lasts longer than 42 weeks. Only five percent of babies arrive on their due dates, and as long as you and your baby are being carefully monitored to ensure good health, you should be able to continue on with your pregnancy until labor occurs naturally. Many first pregnancies especially go past their due dates.

Risks

If your baby is overdue, she may outgrow her environment and this can cause problems. Her head may not engage properly in your pelvis and your cervix may take longer to efface and dilate, making labor more difficult. Placental function may start to decline, resulting in less amniotic fluid around the baby and a lack of nutrients.

Inducing labor

If your baby is thought to be at risk, you will be induced (see page 86) and some hospitals have a policy of induction after a certain time. But sometimes there are no fetal problems; your baby is just not ready to leave her warm and secure environment, or your due date is inaccurate. Due dates are rarely accurate because they are estimated to be around 40 weeks after the start of the last menstrual period although fertilization may occur later than mid month. In such a case, you may like to try and bring on labor naturally. Ways to do this include keeping active, gently stimulating your nipples, which encourages oxytocin to stimulate uterine contractions, or making love frequently. However, doctors disagree over the effectiveness of these techniques.

Kick-count sheet

If there is some cause for concern, you can help to monitor your baby's well-being with a kick-count sheet (see right). Printed forms may be provided by your healthcare provider, but you can also make one yourself with graph paper. Across the top of the paper mark the days of the week for a couple of weeks. Down the side of the paper, mark hours and half hours. Choose a convenient hour twice a day to count the number of movements your baby makes. If your baby makes ten movements within those hours, color in the corresponding square on your graph. If you notice any change or you cannot count ten movements during that time, inform your healthcare provider.

Overdue babies

An overdue baby is called "post-mature" when her environment has started to deteriorate. Depending on how overdue she is, your baby will look rather different from babies born around their expected delivery date. She will probably weigh more and have no vernix covering her body. This can result in her skin peeling. If she had to use some of her fat stores as nourishment, her skin will be wrinkly and baggy—particularly around her abdomen. She may also have very long fingernails and lots of hair on her head.

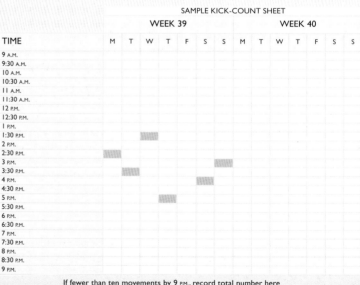

SAMPLE KICK-COUNT SHEET

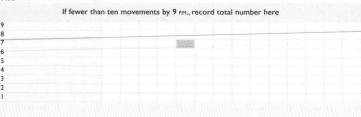

Mom-to-be

First pregnancies generally extend by approximately eight days; another common reason for lateness is the positioning of baby's head. Depending on your health, being one (or even two) weeks overdue should not be considered a cause for concern. While you wait, your healthcare giver may perform some tests to make sure your baby is healthy. These include ultrasound scans to check your baby's size and a "nonstress" test (NST) where your baby's heart-rate is measured. If, however, your pregnancy approaches 42 weeks, your heathcare giver will probably be discussing induction with you.

Baby

If she is still in the uterus your baby is simply putting on weight, and perhaps getting impatient to be born. If she is newborn, she will find that life is very different from in the womb. Fortunately, she is equipped to cope. Now that her lungs have to provide all her oxygen, a major change happens in her heart. Previously there was a hole through the center wall of the heart that allowed blood to bypass the lungs, but when she is born, this hole closes up and blood is diverted through the lungs. She also has instinctive reflexes that serve her well, helping her to feed and to bond with you and your partner.

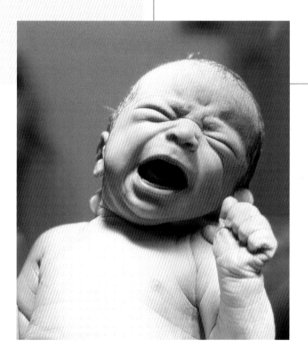

Think about keeping your cell phone turned off should your baby not arrive and you're getting tired of telling people this.

Newborn

Your baby will be cleaned up after birth to remove the remaining vernix, blood, and other fluids covering her.

DATES FOR YOUR DIARY

MONDAY	TUESDAY	WEDNESDAY	THURSDAY	FRIDAY	SATURDAY/SUNDAY

NEWBORN BABY CHECKS

As soon as your baby is born, his umbilical cord will be clamped and cut, and he may be placed onto your stomach or at your breast for you to hold and get to know. You may prefer him to be handed to you cleaned and wrapped up, but immediate skin-to-skin contact helps facilitate the bonding process (see page 68). He will then be examined to determine his health.

The APGAR test
The APGAR was developed in 1952 by obstetric anesthesiologist, Virginia Apgar, and has become a standard tool in assessing newborn babies. It is a series of tests that all babies undergo immediately after birth and then five minutes later, and can be performed while your baby is right next to you. Your baby's heart rate, breathing, muscle tone, color, and reflex actions will be observed and given a score out of ten. A score of seven or more is normal, so if your baby scores less than seven he may need further examination or special assistance.

Standard checks
These checks will usually occur after you and your partner have had some time alone with your baby. In addition to the ones shown here, your baby will be turned onto his stomach and a finger run along his spine to check for signs of spina bifida. His genitals will be checked for abnormalities. His anus will be examined to make sure it has perforated properly.

Your baby's abdomen will be felt to ascertain the size and shape of his internal organs and to check for any obvious protrusions, which are indicative of an umbilical hernia (a surgically repairable congenital malformation).

Your baby's heart and lungs will be examined to make sure they have developed properly and are performing in a satisfactory manner. If you give birth in a hospital or birthing center, before you and your baby leave, a pediatrician will give him a full examination to confirm that he is feeding well, passing stools frequently, and generally progressing healthily.

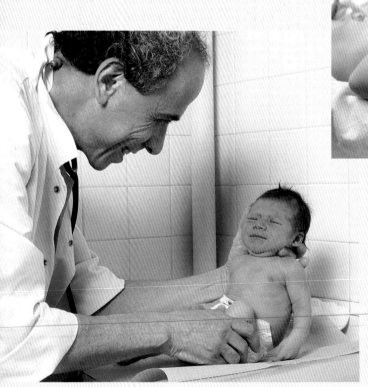

Head and fontanelles
The circumference of his head will be measured and his fontanelles (soft spots on the head) examined. His facial features and inside of his mouth will also be checked for signs of a cleft palate or other defects.

Hips and limbs
Your doctor will bend and circle your baby's legs to make sure there is no hip dislocation. He will also count his fingers and toes.

Mom-to-be

Nearly 10 percent of pregnancies last this long, particularly for first-time mothers, so don't be anxious if you are still carrying. It may even be that your due date was incorrectly calculated, and you are, in fact, running exactly on schedule. You may prefer to attempt to bring labor on naturally by massaging your nipples—or even indulging in a bout of rigorous cleaning—but health professionals disagree about the effectiveness of such techniques. Talk to your doctor about natural and artificial methods of inducing labor (see page 86).

Baby

Your baby is born with a number of important ingrained behaviors, known as neonatal reflexes, many of which are thought to help him survive. If you tickle his cheek, he will turn toward you to find food; if a nipple, pacifier, or finger is put into his mouth, he will suck on it. If you put your finger in his palm, he will grasp it tightly. In fact, so strong is this grasp that you can lift him from a flat surface. If you hold him upright under his arms and let his feet touch the floor, he will appear to walk.

Reflexes

Babies are born with certain reflexes essential to help them cope with life outside the womb. One of the most notable—yet inexplicable— is the grasping reflex.

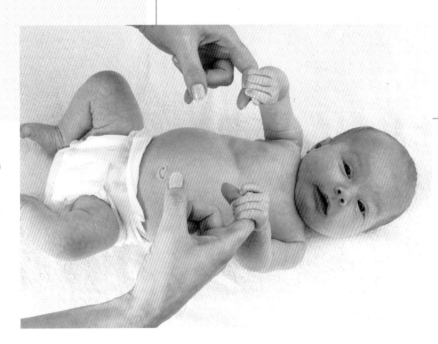

If your baby hasn't been born, you will almost certainly be induced this week.

DATES FOR YOUR DIARY

MONDAY	TUESDAY	WEDNESDAY	THURSDAY	FRIDAY	SATURDAY/SUNDAY

NAMING YOUR BABY

Choosing a name for your baby can be trickier than you think. As well as coming up with something both parents like, the name of your baby will stay with her for the rest of her life, so it must be suitable at all ages.

Choosing a name

As a starting point for discovering which names you like and which you don't, have a look through the numerous baby name books that are available. You should draw up a list of the names you prefer and ask your partner to do the same. Ideally, both of you will have the same name high up on your lists. However, if you have no names in common, perhaps you can find some similar quality. Sometimes a certain consonant (Nicholas, Nina,

Natalie), or a theme such as nature (Holly, Ivy, Lily), or old-fashioned names (George, Mary, Florence), will reappear. If you find a commonality, it will give you both something to build on.

When you decide on a name, make sure it sounds harmonious with your baby's surname. Friends will invariably shorten her name, so think of all the possible diminutives for your chosen name. If you have a strong dislike of any of them, maybe you could use it as a middle name instead. Check that your baby's initials (middle name included) don't spell an unfortunate word or are the same as her brothers and sisters (this could cause confusion), and remember that any trendy names, unusual spellings, or difficult pronunciation might frustrate your baby for the rest of his life! Names are endowed with sounds, symbols, and meanings, and so the name you give your baby may end up playing a great part in defining his personality.

Twin names

Some parents choose names that sound alike, such as Hannah and Anna, but other choices could include names that are anagrams of each other such as May and Amy, or those that have the same meaning but are in different languages such as Zoë (Greek) and Eve (Hebrew) for "life."

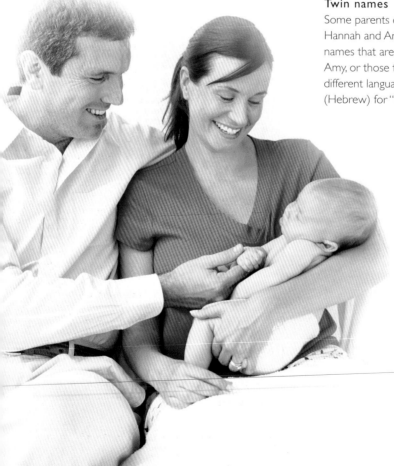

What's in a name

Choose wisely when you give your baby a name. Bear in mind that she will carry her given name not only during her childhood years, but later on in school and throughout her adulthood. She will be known to future generations by the name you give her, so make sure it is something that will suit all the stages of her life.

Middle names

You might want to name your baby after someone in your family or someone you admire from a distance. Although this can be a sign of respect to the person whose name is being used, it can be a problem if your baby grows up to be nothing like that person. Your child may also feel she has to live up to that person's reputation and you may be disappointed if she doesn't. In these instances it is better to use those names as middle names. There has also been a trend recently to use the mother's maiden name, if appropriate, as a middle name. If your baby has brought together different nationalities then you might also like to reflect this cultural ancestry in her middle name.

Meanings

Almost all names have a meaning and many are derived from the Bible. John, one of the oldest names in English history, is a biblical name that means "God has favored" (Jack is a diminutive of it). Others are based on descriptions. Emily has a Germanic derivation and means "industrious" or "eager," while Charles means "a man." Only a few names, Wendy and Vanessa, for example, are invented and have no inherent meaning.

Name inspiration

Some parents name their baby after a favorite city or country—perhaps their honeymoon location (Brooklyn, Sydney, India, Paris)—or a special time or season, such as when baby was conceived (June, Noël, Summer). Other parents use the arts for inspiration. Shakespearean plays, for example, bring to mind Juliet, Olivia, Orlando, and Romeo, while Jane Austen and the Brontës have popularized Emma, Elizabeth, Emily, and Charlotte. Other popular sources include Celtic names such as Megan, Gaelic names such as Aiden, and transferred surnames such as Clifford.

POPULAR BABY NAMES

The top 20 most popular names chosen for babies in the US in 2014 were:

	BOYS		GIRLS
1	Noah	1	Emma
2	Liam	2	Olivia
3	Mason	3	Sophia
4	Jacob	4	Isabella
5	William	5	Ava
6	Ethan	6	Mia
7	Michael	7	Emily
8	Alexander	8	Abigail
9	James	9	Madison
10	Daniel	10	Charlotte
11	Elijah	11	Harper
12	Benjamin	12	Sofia
13	Logan	13	Avery
14	Aiden	14	Elizabeth
15	Jayden	15	Ameila
16	Matthew	16	Evelyn
17	Jackson	17	Ella
18	David	18	Chloe
19	Lucas	19	Victoria
20	Joseph	20	Aubrey

DEVISING A BIRTH PLAN

Writing down all your thoughts about the way you want to give birth can assist you in identifying some important issues. It is also be very helpful to the medical staff if they work shifts in care in the hospital where you give birth. Your birth plan can be written in point form or in paragraphs; what is important is that it briefly outlines your preferences, rather than makes demands. An outline plan is included on page 93. If you prefer not to write your own plan, fill in the blanks on this sample plan. You may change your mind about what you'd like to happen, so photocopy this page before filling it in, and then distribute as necessary.

Before you complete your plan, discuss your ideas with your doctor or nurse-midwife. Their feedback will give you a clearer idea of what is (and is not) feasible. It's important, too, to discuss your plan with your birth partner—and well before the delivery date. This not only helps to involve him or her in the pregnancy and birth but your partner will then be in the best position to help you achieve the birth you want.

After you write your birth plan you should give your partner and other birth attendants a copy. Make sure you

A COPY FOR YOUR CARER

Discuss your birth plan with your doctor or nurse-midwife at least a month before you are due to deliver. Your relationship with your doctor and nurse-midwife is an important one, so it is better to request your preferences, rather than demand them. Give your caregiver a copy of the plan before hospital admittance.

feel confident that they can convey to the medical staff your preferences in the event that you are unable to.

You should also take a copy of your birth plan with you to the hospital so there is a copy of it with your records. Most hospitals have certain policies surrounding birth practices, but they will make an effort to meet your requests. You need to remember, however, that giving birth doesn't always go as planned, so you should be prepared to adapt your plan and to make some on-the-spot decisions during labor and delivery.

Creating your plan
Writing a birth plan can help you understand your options in labor and delivery. Your ideas about birth may change as you progress in your pregnancy, so it's a good idea to revise the plan from time to time.

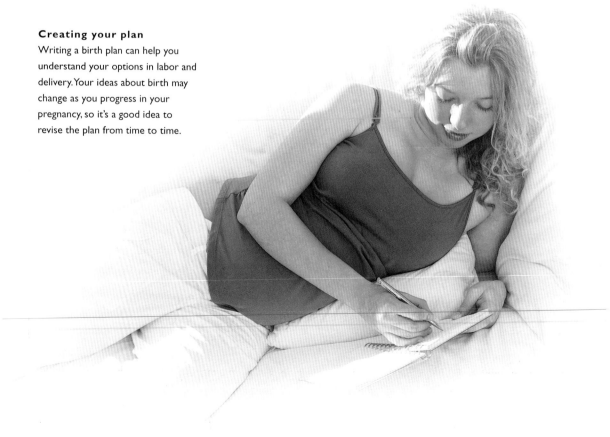

THE BIRTH PLAN OF _____

Where would you like the birth (at home/in hospital or birthing center)?

_____

Do you have any strong feelings about having fetal monitoring (continuous/never, only during certain times, only under certain circumstances)?

_____

What are your requests regarding feeding (breast/bottle, right away, on demand, daytime only)?

_____

How would you like your environment to be (dim lights, music, cushions, or birth stool)?

_____

Do you have any strong feelings about the use of forceps or a vacuum extractor (yes/no, only under certain circumstances)?

_____

How do you feel about the presence of student nurse-midwives or student obstetricians (yes/no)?

_____

Who will be your birth partner or birth assistant? How do you envisage his/her role—present at all times, actively supportive, informed/asked about decisions needing to be made in the event you are unable to?

_____

How would you like your birth to proceed if you need an emergency cesarean section (baby handed to birth partner; type of incision)?

_____

How would you like your baby to be handed to you after the birth (immediately, cleaned and wrapped up, after your partner [if you have a general anesthetic])?

_____

Who should cut the cord, the doctor or nurse-midwife or your birth partner?

_____

Do you have any strong feelings about the placement of your baby while you are recovering (next to you in a crib, in the newborn nursery ward)?

_____

What positions would you prefer to be in during your labor and delivery (sitting upright, squatting, active)?

_____

Do you have any requests if your doctor believes an episiotomy is necessary (would you prefer to risk a tear)?

_____

Do you have a preference for a certain kind of pain relief, such as anesthesia, analgesics, or hydrotherapy, if any?

_____

Would you like the delivery of the placenta to be speeded up artificially (yes/no) and if so, by what method?

_____

YOUR BODY AFTER GIVING BIRTH

Your body will need time to recover from the rigors of labor and/or the trauma of a cesarean section. Eating a healthy diet; engaging in a safe, habitual fitness program, and monitoring your emotions need to be part of the process. Some women prefer to wait until after their postpartum appointment, about six weeks after the birth, before starting a program to get back in shape.

Aches and pains

If you labored, your muscles may ache and you may have strong pains, similar to period pains, in your abdomen. Known as "after pains," these are triggered by the release of oxytocin, the hormone that contracts and shrinks the uterus to decrease bleeding after birth. Happily, the discomfort from postpartum contractions decreases each day and can be lessened by taking safe, painkilling medications such as ibuprofen or acetaminophen.

If you had a vaginal birth, your gential area will be swollen, sore, and stretched. If labor was long and difficult, or you had a tear, stitches, or an episiotomy, you will have pain and discomfort and the perineum (the area between the vagina and anus) may feel quite numb. Try the self-help remedies to help ease the pain.

Lochia

After the birth, blood, mucus, and tissue exit through the uterus. Known as "lochia," this discharge is initially heavy, dark red, and thick and may contain large blood clots. It can be particularly heavy when getting out of bed and breastfeeding. Lochia can last up to six weeks, but gradually the flow becomes less heavy and paler. Use extra-absorbent mentrual pads, not tampons, to absorb the lochia, and change them frequently. If the bleeding suddenly becomes heavier, turns bright red, contains large clots, or smells unpleasant, notify your healthcare provider immediately—it could be a sign of an infection.

Breast discomfort

The hormonal changes that prime your breasts for breastfeeding take place about two to three days after birth, whether you breastfeed or not. Known as "engorgement," your breasts will become larger and firmer and may be painful. To feel more comfortable, it's essential you wear a well-fitting, supportive bra, possibly 24 hours a day, until your milk "comes in" and your breasts soften. Before breastfeeding, you may find it helps to put warm compresses on your breasts; the

SELF HELP FOR PERINEAL PAIN

- Pelvic floor exercises (see page 48) will reduce pain, help you regain muscle tone after delivery, and promote healing by increasing circulation in the area.
- Drinking plenty of fluids dilutes urine so that it doesn't burn as much when you urinate. You should also empty your bladder regularly.
- An ice pack or bag of frozen peas, wrapped in a soft cloth, can be placed on the perineum for 5 minutes, every couple of hours during the first 24 hours.
- Instead of sitting on the toilet seat, squat over it, angling your hips so urine misses the tender spot.
- Keep a pitcher of cool water in the bathroom, so you can pour water between your legs as you urinate and when you have finished so that there is no urine left on your skin.
- Sit in a sitz bath (a bowl filled with warm water) or apply warm compresses for about 20 minutes three times a day.
- Soak a maternity pad in witch hazel; it will cool the area and stop blood from sticking to any pubic hair.

moist heat will dilate the milk ducts making your milk flow more easily.

If you are not going to breastfeed, try putting a cool compress on your breasts and take an analgesic such as acetaminophen or ibuprofen. Don't stimulate your breasts or try to express milk to relieve pressure, because this will only cause your body to produce more milk. Lack of stimulation by a sucking baby will gradually slow and then stop milk production.

If your breasts become inflamed or extremely uncomfortable, see your doctor.

Getting periods back

Periods generally restart within four to six weeks, though if you are breastfeeding, periods may be irregular or not appear until you have stopped. The amount of menstrual flow for the first few cycles can range from scant to very heavy, but should soon settle down into a more consistent pattern after that. Ovulation begins again after the first period following childbirth, so having unprotected sex could result in another pregnancy. To prevent this, some form of contraception is needed as soon as you start having sex again. Breastfeeding mothers may be able to take a progesterone-only pill. Those who are not breastfeeding can start taking birth control pills about two to three weeks after the birth. Barrier contraception should not be used if stitches are present or until the cervix is completely healed.

Elimination difficulties

Although it's essential that the bladder is emptied within six to eight hours of delivery to avoid urinary tract infections and to prevent the bladder from becoming distended, which could cause a loss of muscle tone, some women have no urge to go or want to go but can't. You will probably urinate frequently and copiously about 24 hours after the birth to expel pregnancy fluids. To help get your bladder working, drink plenty of fluids

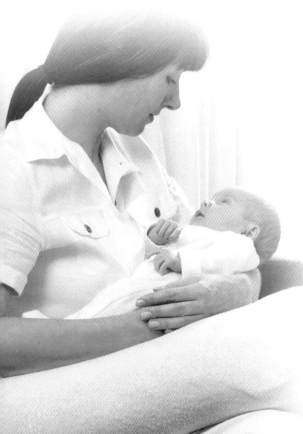

and get up and walk around as soon after the delivery as is allowable.

Although the first few bowel movements may cause discomfort, any stitches won't be affected, and you should be back to normal within a few days. Eating fiber (whole grains and fresh fruit and vegetables) and drinking plenty of fluids will help get your bowels moving again. Gentle exercise and pelvic floor exercises (see page 48) should help to ease any discomfort. If you become constipated, your healthcare provider may suggest stool softeners or a laxative.

Body shape and weight loss

On average, giving birth results in an 11-pound weight loss. Your stomach will stick out due to fluid retention and a distended uterus; your skin will sag because it is overstretched, and you will have lost muscle tone. Over time, your body will get closer to its shape before you gave birth if you eat a healthy, nutritious diet, and make sure you exercise regularly.

Emotional changes

Up to 80 percent of all new mothers suffer from mood changes; vague sadness; feeling weepy, irritable, anxious, and confused—which may occur a day or two after birth and last for about 10 to 14 days. Although the exact cause of "baby blues" or "postpartum blues" is not known, rapid hormone shifts and sleep deprivation are common suspects, which is why you should nap whenever you can and try some relaxation techniques. Despite exhaustion, you may be unable to sleep. Your appetite may rise or fall, or you might feel irritable, nervous, or worried about being a good mother. Rest assured that all such feelings are normal during the first couple of weeks after childbirth. In fact, up to 80 percent of new moms experience them.

The good thing is that the baby blues aren't an illness, and they will go away on their own. No treatment is necessary other than reassurance, support from family and friends, rest, and time.

INDEX